Cardiovascular Disease

Fight It
with
the Blood
Type Diet®

Also by Dr. Peter J. D'Adamo with Catherine Whitney

Eat Right 4 Your Type: The Individualized Diet Solution to Staying Healthy, Living Longer, and Achieving Your Ideal Weight

Cook Right 4 Your Type: The Practical Kitchen Companion to Eat Right 4 Your Type

Live Right 4 Your Type: The Individualized Prescription for Maximizing Health, Metabolism, and Vitality in Every Stage of Your Life

Eat Right 4 Your Type Complete Blood Type Encyclopedia

Eat Right 4 Your Baby: The Individualized Guide to Fertility and Maximum Health During Pregnancy, Nursing, and Your Baby's First Year

Blood Type O: Food, Beverage and Supplement Lists

Blood Type A: Food, Beverage and Supplement Lists

Blood Type B: Food, Beverage and Supplement Lists

Blood Type AB: Food, Beverage and Supplement Lists

Dr. Peter J. D' Adamo's Eat Right 4 (for) Your Type Health Library

Diabetes: Fight It with the Blood Type Diet®

Cancer: Fight It with the Blood Type Diet®

Arthritis: Fight It with the Blood Type Diet®

DR. PETER J. D'ADAMO

WITH CATHERINE WHITNEY

Dr. Peter J. D'Adamo's

Eat Right 4 Your Type

Health Library

Cardiovascular Disease

Fight It with the Blood Type Diet®

G. P. PUTNAM'S SONS

NEW YORK

G. P. Putnam's Sons
Publishers Since 1838
a member of
Penguin Group (USA) Inc.
375 Hudson Street
New York, NY 10014

Library of Congress Cataloging-in-Publication Data

D'Adamo, Peter.
Cardiovascular disease : fight it with the blood type diet /
Peter J. D'Adamo with Catherine Whitney.
p.   cm.—(Eat right 4 (for) your type health library)
Includes index.
ISBN 0-399-15226-1
1. Cardiovascular system—Diseases—Diet therapy.
2. Blood groups.   I. Whitney, Catherine.   II. Title.
RC684.D5D334   2004   2004044391
616.1'0654—dc22

Printed in the United States of America
1   3   5   7   9   10   8   6   4   2

This book is printed on acid-free paper. ∞

DEDICATED TO ALL THE DEVOTED AND
TALENTED RESEARCHERS WHO FOR THE
LAST FIVE DECADES HAVE ENDEAVORED TO
DEEPEN OUR UNDERSTANDING OF THE
IMPORTANT ROLE THE ABO BLOOD
GROUPS PLAY IN THE DEVELOPMENT AND
PREVENTION OF HEART DISEASE

Acknowledgments

THIS BOOK OFFERS THE BEST THAT NATUROPATHIC MEDICINE AND blood type science have to offer in the prevention and treatment of cardiovascular disease. It has been a collaborative process, and I want to express my deep thanks to the people who have been involved in its creation.

I am most grateful to Martha Mosko D'Adamo, not only my partner in life and in parenting but also my partner in bringing the valuable wisdom about blood type to the world. Martha daily provides love, support, insight, and inspiration to all of my endeavors.

Catherine Whitney, my writer, and her partner, Paul Krafin, are invaluable word masters who have once again captured exactly the right tone in tackling this complex topic.

My literary agent and friend, Janis Vallely, always takes time to listen and advise. Her quiet guidance and personal support make the work possible.

I would also like to acknowledge others who have made significant contributions to this book: Heidi Merritt, who continues to make an important contribution to the work; Laura Mittman, N.D., who has selflessly devoted herself to the dream of an Institute for Human Individuality (IfHI); Joseph Pizzorno, N.D., and Jeffrey Bland, Ph.D., for believing in me; John Harris, whose knowledge and careful fact checking have been invaluable; and Catherine's agent, Jane Dystel, who provides support.

Amy Hertz, my editor at Riverhead/Putnam, has been the force behind the success of all the blood type books, and she continues to guide my work with dedication and skill.

As always, I am extremely grateful to the wonderful staff at Riverhead Books and Putnam. They have been tireless and enthusiastic, and their efforts have made it possible to continue bringing this important work to the market.

PETER J. D'ADAMO, N.D.

Contents

Cardiovascular Disease

Fight It
with
the Blood
Type Diet®

New Tools to Fight Cardiovascular Disease

THE BLOOD TYPE DIET CAN BENEFIT EVERYONE. YOU DON'T have to be sick to see the effects. But most of the people who come to my clinic or contact my Web site are dealing with a serious chronic disease or have received a distressing medical diagnosis. They want to know how they can hone the general guidelines of the Blood Type Diet to target their illness. Dr. Peter J. D'Adamo's Eat Right 4 (for) Your Type Health Library has been introduced with these people in mind.

Cardiovascular Disease: Fight It with the Blood Type Diet allows you to take full advantage of the medicinal benefits of eating and living according to your blood type. If you think of the standard Blood Type Diet as the foundation, the guidelines in this book provide a more targeted overlay for people who want to act aggressively to prevent and treat cardiovascular disease. These dietary and lifestyle adaptations, individualized by blood type, supply additional ammunition to your disease-fighting arsenal. Specifically, they can help you improve your cardiovascular fitness, control your blood sugar, achieve a healthy weight, increase your energy and well-being, prevent or manage heart disease, and reduce or eliminate the need for medications and invasive procedures.

Here's what you'll find that's new:

- A disease-fighting category of blood type–specific food values, the **Super Beneficials**, emphasizing foods that have medicinal properties for cardiovascular disease.
- A more detailed breakdown of the **Neutral** category to limit foods that are known to have less nutritional value or can exacerbate your condition. Foods designated **Neutral: Allowed Infrequently** should be minimized or avoided.
- Detailed supplement protocols for each blood type that are calibrated to support you at every stage. They include a **Cardiovascular and Metabolic Enhancement Protocol**, a **Blood Building Protocol**, a **Stress Reduction Protocol**, an **Angina Relief Adjunct**, and a **Surgery Recovery Adjunct**.
- A **4-Week Plan** for getting started that emphasizes what you can do right now to improve your condition and start feeling better right away.
- Plus many strategies for success, quizzes, checklists, and the answers to the questions most frequently asked about cardiovascular disease at my clinic.

The science of blood type continues to provide important clues to the biological and genetic mechanisms that control health and disease. In more than twenty-five years of research and clinical practice, I have successfully treated thousands of patients for hypertension, high cholesterol, insulin resistance, obesity, coronary artery disease, and other cardiovascular conditions. Increasingly, medical doctors and naturopaths throughout the world are applying the blood type principles in their practices, with remarkable results.

I urge you to talk to your physician about the benefits of incorporating individualized, blood type–specific diet, exercise, and lifestyle strategies into your current plan. I am confident that using the guidelines in this book will start you on the road to recovery. Take the step now and use your blood type to your best advantage.

Why Blood
Type Matters

YOU ARE A BIOLOGICAL INDIVIDUAL.

Have you ever wondered why some people are constitutionally frail and susceptible to infection while others seem naturally hardy? Why are some people able to lose weight on a particular diet while others fail? Why do some people age rapidly and show early signs of deterioration while others are full of vitality into their later years?

We are all different. A single drop of your blood contains a biochemical signature as unique to you as your fingerprint. Many of the biochemical differences that make you an individual can be explained by your blood type.

Your blood type influences every facet of your physiology on a cellular level. It has everything to do with how you digest food, your ability to respond to stress, your mental state, the efficiency of your metabolic processes, and the strength of your immune system.

You can greatly improve your health, vitality, and emotional balance by knowing your blood type and by incorporating blood type–specific diet and lifestyle strategies into your health plan.

Be the biochemical individual you were meant to be!

What's Your Blood Type– Cardiovascular Disease Risk?

See what your individualized cardiovascular risk is. Begin with the general risk factors, then go to the specific section related to your blood type.

General Risk Factors

Answer these questions (all blood types)

The following factors are known to contribute to an individual's risk for cardiovascular disease. Answer yes or no to each question, then total the values of the "yes" answers.

RISK FACTOR	Yes	Value
Are you over the age of 60?		1
Is there a history of cardiovascular disease in your family?		2
Are you a smoker?		3
Are you obese (more than 30 pounds overweight)?		3
Do you have high blood pressure?		2
Do you have diabetes (type 1 or type 2)?		2
Do you have a history of heavy alcohol or intravenous drug use?		1
Do you have periodontal (gum) disease?		1
Do you have a history of following very low-calorie "starvation" diets?		1
Total the number of "yes" answer points (16 points maximum)		

BLOOD TYPE–SPECIFIC QUIZZES

The Blood Type O Quiz

The following factors are known to specifically influence Blood Type O's risk for cardiovascular disease. Answer yes or no to each question, then total the values of all "yes" answers.

RISK FACTOR	Yes	Value
Are you a non-secretor? (See page 32.)		3
Is your diet low in fiber (less than 3 to 4 servings per day)?		2
Is your level of aerobic exercise under 4 hours weekly?		3
Do you have thyroid irregularities?		1
Do you suffer from anxiety or depression?		2
Do you have a high-stress job or family environment?		1

RISK FACTOR	Yes	Value
Do you have a triglyceride level over 140 mg/dL?		3
Do you have high cholesterol (overall above 225, and HDL under 45 mg/dL for men and 55 mg/dL for women)?		2
Do you consume a high-starch diet?		2
Total the number of "yes" answer points (19 points maximum)		

Scoring: Total the values of "yes" answer points in each list.

20–35: High to Very High Risk. You are very likely to develop cardiovascular disease, or you already have it. Take immediate action with adherence to the Blood Type Diet, and modify the factors that are in your control.

9–19: Moderate to High Risk. If you make some diet and lifestyle changes and begin an appropriate exercise program, you may avoid cardiovascular disease in the future. Refer to your blood type section to determine which actions you must take.

0–8: Low to Moderate Risk. Your risk for developing cardiovascular disease is relatively low. Keep it that way by adhering to the Blood Type Diet and lifestyle plan.

The Blood Type A Quiz

The following factors are known to specifically influence Blood Type A's risk for cardiovascular disease. Answer yes or no to each question, then total the values of all "yes" answers.

RISK FACTOR	Yes	Value
Are you a non-secretor? (See page 32.)		2
Do you eat red meat?		3
Do you avoid exercise, even stretching or yoga?		2
Do you consume dairy products on a daily basis?		1

RISK FACTOR	Yes	Value
Are your LDL (bad cholesterol) levels over 110mg/dL?		2
Do you have a high stress job or family environment?		2
Do you have a triglyceride level over 150 mg/dL?		2
Do you have high cholesterol (overall above 200, and HDL under 45 mg/dL for men and 55 mg/dL for women)?		4
Do you often have trouble sleeping, and wake feeling tired?		1
Total the number of "yes" answer points (19 points maximum)		

Scoring: Total the values of YES answer points in each list.

20–35: High to Very High Risk. You are very likely to develop cardiovascular disease, or you already have it. Take immediate action with adherence to the Blood Type Diet, and modify the factors that are in your control.

9–19: Moderate to High Risk. If you make some diet and lifestyle changes and begin an appropriate exercise program, you may avoid cardiovascular disease in the future. Refer to your blood type section to determine which actions you must take.

0–8: Low to Moderate Risk. Your risk for developing cardiovascular disease is relatively low. Keep it that way by adhering to the Blood Type Diet and lifestyle plan.

The Blood Type B Quiz

The following factors are known to specifically influence Blood Type B's risk for cardiovascular disease. Answer yes or no to each question, then total the values of all "yes" answers.

RISK FACTOR	Yes	Value
Are you a non-secretor? (See page 32.)		2
Do you consume a high-starch diet?		2
Do you eat chicken or corn-derived products?		2
Are your LDL (bad cholesterol) levels over 110mg/dL?		3
Do you suffer from anxiety or depression?		1
Is you total weekly exercise time under four hours?		3
Do you have a triglyceride level over 160 mg/dL?		2
Do you have high cholesterol (overall above 210, and HDL under 55 mg/dL for men and 60 mg/dL for women)?		2
Do you often have trouble sleeping, and wake feeling tired?		2
Total the number of "yes" answer points (19 points maximum)		

Scoring: Total the values of "yes" answer points in each list.

20–35: High to Very High Risk. You are very likely to develop cardiovascular disease, or you already have it. Take immediate action with adherence to the Blood Type Diet, and modify the factors that are in your control.

5–19: Moderate to High Risk. If you make some diet and lifestyle changes and begin an appropriate exercise program, you may avoid cardiovascular disease in the future. Refer to your blood type section to determine which actions you must take.

0–8: Low to Moderate Risk. Your risk for developing cardiovascular disease is relatively low. Keep it that way by adhering to the Blood Type Diet and lifestyle plan.

The Blood Type AB Quiz

The following factors are known to specifically influence Blood Type AB's risk for cardiovascular disease. Answer yes or no to each question, then total the values of all "yes" answers.

RISK FACTOR	Yes	Value
Are you a non-secretor? (See page 32.)		1
Do have a high-stress job or family environment?		2
Do you eat chicken or corn-derived products?		2
Are your LDL (bad cholesterol) levels over 110mg/dL?		3
Do you suffer from anxiety or depression?		1
Is you total weekly exercise time under four hours?		3
Do you have a triglyceride level over 160 mg/dL?		2
Do you have high cholesterol (overall above 200, and HDL under 55 mg/dL for men and 60 mg/dL for women)?		3
Do you often have trouble sleeping, and wake feeling tired?		2
Total the number of "yes" answer points (19 points maximum)		

Scoring: Total the values of "yes" answer points in each list.

20–35: High to Very High Risk. You are very likely to develop cardiovascular disease, or you already have it. Take immediate action with adherence to the Blood Type Diet, and modify the factors that are in your control.

9–19: Moderate to High Risk. If you make some diet and lifestyle changes and begin an appropriate exercise program, you may avoid cardiovascular disease in the future. Refer to your blood type section to determine which actions you must take.

0–8: Low to Moderate Risk. Your risk for developing cardiovascular disease is relatively low. Keep it that way by adhering to the Blood Type Diet and lifestyle plan.

PART I

Blood Type
and
Cardiovascular
Disease:
A Basic Primer

The Genesis of Cardiovascular Disease

THE STUDY OF BLOOD TYPES HAS LED TO AN IMPORTANT breakthrough in the way we must view cardiovascular disease. Although the health of the cardiovascular system depends on a complex blend of many factors, including diet, exercise, stress, and the effects of other diseases, we now understand that a very important component involves genetics—including the genetics of blood type.

Your blood type can influence the workings of your cardiovascular system in several ways. For example, there is a particularly strong correlation between blood type and the ability to metabolize dietary fats and oils. Blood type has been shown to directly influence the viscosity (thickness) of the blood, which has powerful implications with regard to circulation. The different ABO blood types have varying levels of "normal" cholesterol in the blood, and blood type also influences the reactivity of the blood vessel walls—allowing for attachment of white blood cells and the subsequent inflammation that we now know is crucial to artery damage.

Blood type genetics also plays a role in your chemical response to stress. Since stress is an important risk factor for heart disease, the blood type–specific variations in the response to stress can become a key factor in cardiac health.

Of course, not every risk factor for heart disease has a blood type component. For example, a nutrient-poor diet or smoking will increase your odds of developing cardiovascular disease, no matter what your blood type. The bottom line is that there are several pathways to the heart, and several pathways, too, to heart disease. Knowledge of the dynamics is preventive power.

The Key to Your Heart

ARISTOTLE BELIEVED that the heart was the seat of the soul, and, indeed, it has maintained a metaphorical eminence in art and poetry. This core of our beings weighs a mere ten and a half ounces, is hollow, and measures about the size of a human fist. This is not very big when you consider the job it does. In some animals, such as horses, the size of the heart is much greater. The heart is also bigger in champion endurance athletes, due to genetics and training. Each day, your heart beats over 100,000 times and pumps about 2,000 gallons of blood, enough to fill a petrol tanker. In a seventy-year lifetime, an average human heart beats more than 2.5 billion times. It has been speculated that the life span of any species is relative to the absolute number of heartbeats over the course of its life: Smaller-sized, short-lived species have very high heart rates, while larger, longer-lived species have heart rates that are much slower.

In a sense, your heart is really two hearts—the left heart and the right. Both sides pump the same amount of blood, but to different locations of the body, and at different pressures. The right ventricle pumps blood to your lungs, where gases such as carbon dioxide are removed and oxygen is added. This is a short trip and requires little pressure development, so the right ventricle is rather thin walled, like a fireplace bellows. The left ventricle is the real workhorse, pumping oxygenated blood that has returned from the lungs to the entire body.

That means moving blood through an incredible maze of blood vessels at great pressure. The left heart muscle is thicker as a result.

Your circulatory system, composed of heart and blood vessels, contains five quarts of blood. Your heart pumps these five quarts through 60,000 miles of veins and arteries. The round-trip takes about one minute, and sometimes the blood reaches a speed of ten miles per hour.

Your heart is an amazingly resilient organ. Alexis Carrel, the famous experimental biologist who received the 1912 Nobel Prize in Physiology or Medicine, concluded that, given an optimum supply of nutrients and oxygen, the heart is capable of functioning perfectly for over two centuries. The most common forms of heart disease do not result from a wearing-out of the heart but rather from a breakdown in the supply of nutrients, usually the result of disease in the arteries upon which the heart relies.

Atherosclerosis: Narrowing of the Arteries

MOST PROBLEMS with the heart stem from narrowing of the coronary arteries. The process begins with the development of fatty streaks along the walls of major blood vessels and the formation of plaque from cholesterol and calcium. These cause obstructions that prevent the free flow of blood. This condition is termed atherosclerosis (*athero*, from the Greek word for "gruel" or "fat," and *sclerosis*, from the Greek word for "hard"). Atherosclerosis can affect large- and medium-sized arteries; the specific kind of artery and the location of the plaque vary with each person. Atherosclerosis is a slow, progressive disease that may take its toll over a period of decades. Often, it doesn't noticeably affect people until they are in their fifties or sixties. It is a sobering thought that early signs of atherosclerosis, such as fatty streaks or lipid deposits, are sometimes found in the aortas of children as young as three years old.

It is unknown exactly how atherosclerosis begins or what causes it, although some scientists believe that initiation occurs when the innermost layer of the artery, called the endothelium, becomes damaged. In addition to genetics and lifestyle, an increasingly recognized trigger point for cardiovascular disease is chronic, low-grade infection. Infections with chlamydia, *Helicobacter pylori,* chronic bronchitis, and frequent dental infections and gum disease have been linked to elevated serum levels of an inflammatory modulator called C-reactive protein, and have been implicated as risk factors for cardiovascular disease. Elevated serum levels of C-reactive protein can also be detected in the presence of chronic low-grade systemic inflammation.

It may well be that the genesis of cardiovascular disease lies with an immunologic event, such as an infection, with its further development dependent on other risk factors, such as elevated cholesterol. Other risk factors may themselves be dependent on an initiating event, such as damage to the artery lining from a chronic infection.

Other means of initiating damage to the arterial wall include the effects of superoxide free radicals, which react with the delicate lining. Smoking, for example, dramatically increases the activity of free radicals. Regardless of the original provocation, fats, cholesterol, fibrin, platelets, cellular debris, and calcium are deposited in the arterial wall over time. These substances can stimulate the cells of the arterial wall to produce still other substances that result in further accumulation of cells causing atherosclerotic lesions, called plaque. Plaque may partially or totally block the blood's flow through an artery, causing bleeding into the plaque or formation of a blood clot (thrombus) on the plaque's surface. If either of these occurs and blocks the entire artery, a heart attack or stroke may occur.

Contributing Factors

THERE ARE MANY conditions that exist in relationship to cardiovascular disease. Individually or in combination, they can provoke heart attacks, strokes, or heart failure.

Hypertension

Hypertension, or chronic high blood pressure, is associated with heart disease, stroke, congestive heart failure, vision impairment, and kidney disease. It is famously known as the silent killer, as there are usually no obvious signs of its presence.

Diabetes

Cardiovascular disease is the leading cause of death among diabetics and is closely linked with other factors, such as high cholesterol, high blood pressure, and high triglycerides. People with diabetes often have high cholesterol and/or high triglycerides. Your body uses cholesterol to build cell walls and to produce certain vitamins and hormones. Your body uses triglycerides as stored fat. Stored fat keeps you warm, protects your body's organs, and gives you energy reserves. When lipids are out of control, they collect and harden into arterial plaque, which blocks the flow of blood to the heart.

Normal Blood Pressure	Less than 120/80
Pre-Hypertension	120/80 to 139/89
Mild Hypertension	140/90 to 159/99
Moderate Hypertension	160/100 to 179/109
Severe Hypertension	180/110 and above

**THE HEALTHIEST
BLOOD FAT LEVELS ARE**

Total cholesterol under 200 mg/dL
LDL cholesterol under 130 mg/dL
HDL cholesterol over 35 mg/dL
Triglycerides under 200 mg/dL
Extrapolate these numbers according to blood type variations identified in the quizzes.

Metabolic Syndrome

Metabolic conditions often occur simultaneously. In recent years, medical researchers have given increasing attention to a condition they refer to as metabolic syndrome (formerly Syndrome X). Metabolic syndrome, which affects about 47 million Americans, is a clustering of problems that together form a dangerous and potentially deadly state. These conditions include insulin resistance, high blood sugar, elevated triglycerides, high LDL (low-density lipoproteins) cholesterol, low HDL (high-density lipoproteins) cholesterol, high blood pressure, and obesity (especially abdominal fat). Metabolic syndrome is the gateway to heart disease. Most diabetics have at least one or two additional conditions and need to monitor them to reduce the risk of heart disease.

Metabolic Syndrome Involves at Least Three of the Following:

- Waist more than 40 inches around in men or 35 inches in women.
- Triglyceride levels of 150 or greater.
- HDL, or "good" cholesterol, less than 40 in men or less than 50 in women.
- Blood pressure of 130/85 or more.
- Fasting blood sugar of 100 or more.

Blood Pumping Disorders

There are several conditions that interfere with blood flow to the heart. Often they are associated with larger chronic conditions, such as coronary artery disease or peripheral artery disease. They include:

- **Congestive Heart Failure** This includes any condition that disturbs the pumping of blood through the heart muscle and throughout the body, or prevents blood from oxygenating the lungs. This backup of blood creates a fluid buildup in the lungs. There are many symptoms of this condition including weakness, fatigue, shortness of breath, and edema.

- **Atrial Arrhythmias** Our hearts pump blood throughout our bodies using an extraordinary electrical mechanism. When that electrical mechanism misfires, atrial fibrillation occurs. The atrium is the receiving chamber for blood coming to the heart. Atrial fibrillation means that the heart rhythm has been disturbed—an arrhythmia has occurred—and that the chambers of the heart are no longer contacting in their usual organized manner. Because of this, the lower chambers of the heart—the ventricles—begin to quiver rapidly and irregularly. This dangerous state can lead to heart failure and death.

- **Ventricular Arrhythmias** This is a disturbance of the electrical rhythm of the more muscular of the heart's pumping stations, the one that distributes the blood throughout the rest of the body. Ventricular fibrillation refers to a breakdown of the heart's electrical mechanism, its rhythm center. Instead of contracting in its usual way, an arrhythmia occurs, and the heart begins quivering. Ventricular arrhythmia is a life-threatening condition, and someone in this state must receive defibrillation within minutes to avoid complete heart failure and death.

- **Aneurysms** There are many forms of aneurysms possible. The term refers to the weakening and possible rupture of a blood vessel or arterial wall. Aneurysms can go undetected for years, and when they erupt they can be fatal.

Stroke: A Cerebrovascular Accident

A STROKE IS LIKE a heart attack to the brain. It occurs when an artery that supplies blood to the brain bursts or is blocked by a blood clot. An ischemic stroke is caused by a blocked or narrowed artery. A hemor-

Angina Pectoris: Chest Pain

Angina pectoris is a recurring pain or discomfort in the chest that occurs when some part of the heart does not receive enough blood. It is a common symptom of coronary heart disease, which occurs when vessels that carry blood to the heart become narrowed and blocked due to atherosclerosis. An episode of angina is not a heart attack. Angina pain means that some of the heart muscle is not getting enough blood temporarily—for example, during exercise, when the heart has to work harder. The pain does not mean that the heart muscle is suffering irreversible, permanent damage. Episodes of angina seldom cause permanent damage to the heart muscle but serve as a warning that there are serious problems with the coronary artery circulation.

rhagic stroke develops when an artery in the brain leaks or bursts and causes bleeding inside the brain tissue or near the surface of the brain.

There is usually little advance warning of a stroke. Symptoms begin suddenly and may include a numbness, weakness, or paralysis of the face, arm, or leg, especially on one side of the body; blurred vision; dizziness or confusion; or a blinding headache.

Strokes usually occur in the elderly. More than 66 percent of all strokes happen after age sixty-five. They are typically linked with other chronic cardiovascular conditions. High blood pressure is the leading risk factor for stroke after age 65. Circulation problems common to advanced stages of diabetes can also trigger a stroke. About 25 percent of people with diabetes die of stroke. Heart disease itself places an individual at greater risk for stroke. Weakening of arterial walls, the development of blood clots, and damage to the heart muscle all contribute to the potential for a stroke.

Know Your Risks

CORONARY HEART DISEASE is related to a number of risk factors, including high blood pressure, high blood cholesterol, smoking, obesity, and physical inactivity—all of which can be controlled. Problems arise when we try to portray risk factors as being identical for entirely different groups of people. It is here that many of the recent assertions about the connections between lifestyle and cardiovascular disease begin to break down. While many people do fit the official risk factor profile for heart disease, equally large numbers do not. Genetic factors, such as blood type, provide an extra level of interpretation, identifying the biomarkers that can show who will suffer from cardiovascular disease because of one factor and who will develop the disease for an entirely different reason. Risk factors are conditions that increase your chances of developing heart disease. Some can be changed and some cannot. Although these factors each increase the risk of cardiovascular disease, they do not describe all the causes. Even with no recognized risk factors some people still develop heart problems.

There is a very distinct difference among the blood types with regard to their incidence of heart disease. Though largely unnoticed by the conventional medical authorities, the literature documenting a link between blood type and heart disease is extensive and compelling.

The Blood Type– Cardiovascular Disease Connection

IT MAKES GOOD SENSE TO LOOK FOR DIFFERENT CAUSES OF action in different people, since the evidence is so strong that there are substantial variations among heart disease sufferers. While each blood type can develop elements of cardiovascular disease, each appears to do so for different reasons. When you understand your individual risk factors for cardiovascular disease, in light of your blood type, you gain new control over your health. Although you cannot change your blood type, you can make appropriate alterations in your diet and lifestyle that will greatly reduce your risks.

The Cholesterol Paradox

UNDOUBTEDLY THE MOST controversial aspect of the Blood Type Diet has been the use of animal-derived proteins for Blood Types O and B. The conventional argument is that high-protein diets cannot be heart healthy since they are high in cholesterol.

Simple explanations for deadly health conditions are always very seductive. Yet by posing this rigid standard for heart health, conventional medicine ignores individual variations that can significantly influence one's potential for disease.

According to the National Institutes of Health's own statistics, about one-third of heart attacks occur in people over age eighty. In about half of these cases, the victims have normal blood cholesterol levels. Of the remaining heart attack victims, only half have a modifiable risk factor, such as smoking, high blood pressure, or high cholesterol. The others have no recognizable risk factors. They exercise, do not smoke, are not overweight, and have normal blood pressure and cholesterol. Using this measure, only about 10 to15 percent of heart attacks can be prevented by lowering blood cholesterol.

There are countless studies of populations whose dietary makeup defies all conventional wisdom about cholesterol and heart disease. Notably, these populations are almost exclusively Blood Type O, with some Blood Type B, and most of them have long traditions of being carnivores as opposed to agrarians. For example, the people of the Samburu tribe of Africa, along with several other tribes of central Kenya and the Rift Valley, consume approximately a pound of meat and a couple of gallons of raw milk every day as their main diet. This is double the amount of animal fat in the average American diet, yet the average cholesterol levels (about 170 mg/dL) in these tribes are lower than those of the majority of Americans.

Somalian shepherds tending herds of camel subsist almost entirely on camel milk, which is much fattier than cow's milk. The average person consumes about six quarts every day, containing approximately a pound or more of butter fat. Sixty percent of the diet is animal fat, yet cholesterol levels average a strikingly low 150 mg/dL.

The Masai people of Kenya revel in the milk of their native Zebu cattle and gorge regularly on its meat. In spite of this, cholesterol levels among the Masai are the lowest measured worldwide, a mere half of the American average.

The native Inuits of Greenland have very low rates of coronary artery disease. This is usually attributed to seafood diets high in omega-3 polyunsaturated fatty acids. It is a little-known fact, however, that this group has among the world's highest percentage of Blood Type O individuals. Approximately 98 percent of the population is Blood Type O.

Considering these facts, the question becomes: Which individuals can modify their risk factors by lowering cholesterol, and which should emphasize other factors?

If we are serious about halting the course of coronary artery disease, along with related diseases such as hypertension and diabetes, we must look beyond simplistic solutions. The study of blood types has led to one important breakthrough in this effort. Simply put, depending on your blood type, you may have vastly different risk factors for heart disease. Furthermore, your blood type affects the course of treatment and survival once you do have heart disease.

Extensive study references on the relationship between blood type and cardiovascular disease are available on our Web site— www.dadamo.com—and in the books *Live Right 4 Your Type* and *Eat Right 4 Your Type Complete Blood Type Encyclopedia.*

Blood Types A and AB: The Blood Type–Cholesterol Factor

A NUMBER OF STUDIES show that Blood Types A and AB are more likely to be at risk of heart disease by virtue of elevated cholesterol.

- The relationship between blood type and total serum cholesterol levels was examined in a Japanese population to determine whether elevated cholesterol levels are associated with Blood Type A, as has been demonstrated in many West European populations. The results showed that cholesterol levels were very significantly elevated in Blood Type A compared to the other blood types.

- A study examining a total of 380 marker/risk factor combinations found associations between Blood Type A and both total serum cholesterol and LDL cholesterol, while elevated cholesterol was not found to be associated with a greater risk for Blood Type B.

- A Hungarian study measured the cholesterol of 653 patients who underwent coronary angiography between 1980 and 1985 at the Hungarian Institute of Cardiology. The results showed that Blood Type A was more frequent and Blood Type O was less frequent than normally seen in the Hungarian population. Differences were also observed between the blood types in the areas of the vessels where the narrowing of the coronary arteries had occurred.

Several forms of elevated lipoproteins are inherited. One of the more common forms of hyperlipoproteinaemia is called IIb and is characterized by increased LDL and VLDL (*very* bad cholesterol). It results in premature hardening of the arteries, obstruction of the carotid artery (the artery that supplies blood to the head and brain), peripheral artery disease, heart attack, and stroke. Since all of these disorders show higher rates of occurrence in Blood Type A, it is not surprising that studies have found a significant connection between a hyperlipoproteinaemia IIb and Blood Type A in both newborns and in patients who have suffered heart attacks.

Blood Types O and B: The Carbohydrate Intolerance Factor

FOR BLOOD TYPES O and B, the leading risk factor for heart disease is not so much the fat in the food as the fat on the person. And in this case, the elevated risk factor is due to carbohydrate intolerance. When Blood Types O and B adopt low-fat diets rich in metabolically inactivating lectins—foods that aren't right for their type—they gain weight.

This particular kind of weight gain is a major risk factor for heart disease.

For many years, heart experts have been saying that high triglycerides are not an independent risk for heart disease but are only dangerous in combination with other factors. However, increasing evidence points to elevated triglycerides as a risk factor on their own, and this partially explains the anomaly of the Blood Types O and B pathway to heart disease.

Triglycerides are formed by three fatty chains linked to one another. Most fat in food and the human body exists in this form. Diabetics often have high triglyceride levels, and diabetes is believed to be the leading cause of hypertriglyceridemia. In other words, insulin resistance, caused by carbohydrate intolerance, leads to high triglycerides.

A classic sign of insulin resistance is the "apple-shaped figure," characterized by a broad girth at the midsection. Fat cells located in the abdomen release fat into the blood more easily than fat cells found elsewhere. For example, "pear-shaped" individuals, with fat located in the hips and thighs, do not have the same health risks. The release of fat from the abdomen begins within three to four hours after a meal is consumed, compared to many more hours for other fat cells. This easy release shows up as higher triglycerides and free fatty acid levels. Free fatty acids cause insulin resistance, and elevated triglycerides usually coincide with low HDL ("good" cholesterol), making abdominal fat a precursor of cardiovascular problems. Overproduction of insulin as a result of insulin resistance syndrome has also been shown to increase the production of very bad cholesterol (VLDL).

At long last the medical establishment is beginning to recognize the need to step outside of its narrow box and expand its thinking regarding cardiovascular risk factors. Although there is ample evidence that cholesterol plays an important role in atherosclerosis and heart disease for some people, it is also clear that a large number of people do not fit this limited profile.

Blood Types O and B: Cholesterol Protection

THERE IS A physiological explanation for the relative protection Blood Types O and B enjoy from high-protein diets. Intestinal alkaline phosphatase, an enzyme manufactured in the small intestine, which has the primary function of splitting dietary cholesterol and fats, is naturally high in these blood types—especially secretors. Conversely, Blood Types A and AB have lower levels of this enzyme. Studies suggest that this inability to break down dietary fat in part predisposes Blood Types A and AB to higher cholesterol and more heart attacks. Conversely, Blood Types O and B are somewhat protected by their ability to break down dietary fat.

Intestinal alkaline phosphatase activity rises following the ingestion of a fat-containing meal, especially if the fat is saturated (i.e., mostly derived from animal protein). In a study of volunteers given different test meals, the after-meal rise in serum intestinal alkaline phosphatase activity was significantly greater following the high-protein meal than following the lower-protein meal, and significantly higher in Blood Types O and B. It appears that intestinal alkaline phosphatase gives these blood types metabolic advantages when they eat high-protein meals. In fact, the consumption of protein further increases the levels of alkaline phosphatase in their intestines. Without protein in their diets, they do not gain the benefits of the specialized fat-busting enzymes in their intestines. This explains why Blood Types O and B can lower their cholesterol by adopting high-protein diets.

Recently, an intriguing study helped to cast some light on why Blood Types A and AB have such low levels of alkaline phosphatase activity. In an article entitled "Intestinal Alkaline Phosphatase and the ABO Blood Group System—A New Aspect," researchers presented evidence that the A antigen may itself inactivate alkaline phosphatase. They speculated that the lower levels of this enzyme, and the subsequent inability to break down dietary fats, may actually be a physical expression of the A antigen. The authors found that the red cells of Blood Types A and AB bind almost all intestinal alkaline phosphatase, while the red cells of Blood Types O and B do so to a much lesser degree.

Blood Type–Mediated Stress Factors

CHRONIC STRESS, caused by sleep deprivation, overwork, emotional distress, pain, or any number of external and internal factors, appears to increase the risk of heart disease. Stress can exacerbate other risk factors, such as overeating, smoking, and high blood pressure. Stress can trigger the release of hormones that promote blood clots. Stress releases fatty acids and glucose into the bloodstream. These can be converted into natural fat and cholesterol and deposited on arterial walls. Such deposits create resistance to the blood flow through the arteries and contribute to high blood pressure.

Differences between blood types with regard to stress chemistry may account for some of the observed differences in heart disease victims that appear to be linked to blood type.

Blood Type and Blood Flow

THERE ARE DIFFERENCES among the blood types when it comes to blood clotting factors. Blood Types A and AB have more easily clotting blood, and Blood Types O and B have blood that does not clot as easily. This is a critical distinction—indeed, it can be a matter of life or death. When blood vessels are cut or damaged, the loss of blood from the system must be stopped before shock and possible death occur. This is accomplished by solidification of the blood, a process called coagulation, or clotting.

Your bloodstream contains special nonliving components called platelets, which are responsible for your blood's clotting abilities. Basically, a blood clot consists of a plug of platelets enmeshed in a network of insoluble protein molecules called fibrin. Platelet aggregation and fibrin formation both require the enzyme thrombin. Clotting also requires calcium, which is why blood banks use a chelating agent to bind the calcium in donated blood so it will not clot in the bag.

There are at least a dozen other protein clotting factors, and most of these circulate in your blood as inactive enzyme precursors. A bleeding disorder, such as hemophilia, occurs when one or more of these clotting factors is missing.

Blood type influences one of the more important clotting factors, called factor VIII. Studies dating back to the 1960s have repeatedly shown that a deficiency in factor VIII is linked to Blood Type O, and to a lesser extent Blood Type B, while Blood Types A and AB apparently have higher than average amounts of factor VIII. So the blood of Blood Types A and AB tends to clot more readily than that of Blood Types O and B.

Unlike the other clotting factors, factor VIII is not an enzyme. It normally circulates in the plasma bound to von Willebrand Factor (vWF). Both are serum proteins. When thrombin is activated by injury to the vessel wall, it chops factor VIII free from von Willebrand Factor and activates it. Von Willebrand Factor goes on to bind to the ruptured blood vessel surface, where it stimulates platelets to stick together. The active factor VIII (now called factor VIIIa) reacts with another factor (factor IXa) and calcium to help localize the site of clot formation to the injured vessel.

High levels of factor VIII have been linked to coronary artery disease, and this may in part explain why coronary artery disease shows a higher rate of occurrence in Blood Types A and AB. For example, there is evidence that hemophiliacs experience less coronary artery disease than average, so high factor VIII levels may contribute to the incidence of coronary artery disease by increasing one's potential for developing blood clots.

Blood Types A and AB, with a greater tendency for blood clots, are more likely to suffer from strokes caused by blockages and have a higher overall risk of ischemic strokes, which are caused by blocked or narrowed arteries. Blood Types O and B, with thinner blood, may be more at risk for hemorrhagic strokes, which occur when an artery in the brain leaks or bursts and causes bleeding inside the brain tissue or near the surface of the brain.

Intermittent Claudication

THE WORD CLAUDICATION comes from the Latin *claudicare*, meaning to limp. Intermittent claudication is a condition characterized by an aching, crampy, tired, and sometimes burning pain in the legs that comes and goes. It typically occurs with walking and goes away with rest. In very severe claudication, the pain is also felt at rest. Intermittent claudication is caused by poor circulation of blood in the arteries of the legs. It may occur in one or both legs, and often worsens over time. However, some people complain only of weakness in the legs when walking, or a feeling of "tiredness" in the buttocks. A related condition, venous claudication, results from inadequate venous drainage. There are significantly higher rates of intermittent claudication in Blood Type A individuals, and to some extent in Blood Type AB individuals, when compared to other non-A blood types.

Inflammatory Effects

ONE REASON SO many forms of cardiovascular disease are more frequently seen in Blood Type A individuals may be related to the role of selectins. Selectins are cell-to-cell molecules involved in the adhesion of white blood cells to the blood vessel walls—a function that is part of the immune system's response to fighting infection. Improperly controlled, selectins can over-respond, causing increased inflammation on the blood vessel walls, which is now known to be a factor in some heart disease. Elevated levels of certain selectins are linked with Blood Type A.

Secretor Status Matters

ALTHOUGH EVERYONE CARRIES a blood type antigen on their blood cells, about 80 percent of the population also secretes blood type antigens into body fluids, such as saliva, mucus, and sperm. These people are called secretors. The 20 percent of the population that does not secrete blood type antigens into body fluids are called non-secretors.

Since blood type antigens are crucial to metabolic function and immune defense, being unable to secrete them into body fluids can place non-secretors at a disadvantage. In general, non-secretors are far more likely to suffer from cardiovascular disease and related syndromes. Extensive research into the effect of secretor status on disease shows the following:

- Non-secretors of all blood types have lower levels of intestinal alkaline phosphatase activity than secretors. It has been estimated that the serum alkaline phosphatase activity of non-secretors is only about 20 percent of that of secretors. As a result, non-secretors have more difficulty splitting dietary cholesterol and fats and should eat less animal protein than secretors.
- Non-secretors of all blood types are reported to have shorter bleeding times and a tendency toward higher factor VIII and von Willebrand Factor, predisposing them to arterial clots.
- Non-secretors of all blood types have a higher risk of myocardial infarction (heart attack) than secretors.
- Non-secretors of all blood types are at a greater risk of developing type 2 diabetes, a major risk factor for developing cardiovascular disease.
- Non-secretors of all blood types are more likely to have metabolic syndrome, a group of metabolic problems comprised of insulin resistance, elevated LDL cholesterol, elevated triglycerides, high blood pressure, and obesity. This cluster of metabolic disorders seems to promote the development of type 2 diabetes, atherosclerosis, and cardiovascular disease.

Since secretor status is a critical factor in preventing and treating cardiovascular disease, the individualized Blood Type Diet plans include variations based on secretor status.

For more information about health factors associated with your secretor status, refer to *Live Right 4 Your Type* and *Eat Right 4 Your Type Complete Blood Type Encyclopedia.*

Fighting Cardiovascular Disease with Conventional and Blood Type Therapies

THE BLOOD TYPE DIET IS A CENTRAL ADJUNCT TO YOUR cardiovascular disease battle plan. Your individualized blood type strategy will help you to maximize your disease-fighting capabilities and permit you to vigorously wage war against the particular form of cardiovascular disease you have developed.

If you are currently under medical supervision for a cardiovascular condition, have had a heart attack, angioplasty, or heart bypass surgery; and/or are taking medications to control cholesterol, blood pressure, angina, or diabetes, the diet and lifestyle guidelines specified for your blood type can provide an excellent support system. Most of my patients use the best treatments that conventional medicine has to offer, along with the added benefits of a diet that is genetically suited to their needs.

Conventional Treatment Protocols

THERE ARE MANY new treatments for cardiovascular disease currently in the pipeline at top research facilities and pharmaceutical laboratories throughout the world. These treatments run the gamut from a synthetic of large-molecule HDL that acts as a kind of "drano" for the arteries, sweeping plaque from their walls, to cutting-edge genetic research that may someday allow new arteries and organs to be grown from an individual's own stem cells. Experimental treatments are currently being conducted using dual pressure cuffs on patients' legs to push more blood under pressure into diseased hearts and forcing ancillary veins to be formed and grown. With regular exercise, the ancillary veins remain functional, providing increased blood flow to the heart, naturally bypassing blocked or narrowed arteries. If successful, these treatments might allow previously disabled patients to receive relief from angina and shortness of breath.

The following are the most common treatments currently being used to treat cardiovascular disease.

Medications

There are several classes of medicines used to treat conditions associated with cardiovascular disease. There is no question that many of them are very effective. However, it is also clear that individuals differ. Not every patient will respond similarly to a drug. It is up to the patient to be proactive when a medication is prescribed—to consider all of the factors, pro and con, before beginning a course of treatment. Certainly, blood type is a significant factor. While I would not presume to make a blanket statement that specific heart medicines should be avoided by certain blood types, I would urge you to ask your doctor to consider your blood type–specific tendencies, especially regarding blood clotting factors, cholesterol and triglyceride levels, and risk factors for heart attack.

Statins: A powerful new weapon against LDL cholesterol (the "bad" cholesterol) was introduced in the battle against cardiovascular disease in the late 1980s. It wasn't until 1994 that a large research study found that statins dramatically reduced deaths from heart attack and stroke. Large numbers of people are now taking one of the major statins currently available. Although some people experience unpleasant side effects—nausea, digestive discomfort, muscle weakness—most tolerate the drugs exceptionally well, and the market continues to grow as millions of people are prescribed cholesterol-lowering statin drugs. For those patients with high cholesterol levels, the statins have been effective in lowering total cholesterol numbers. Recent findings indicate the statins may also play a major role in preventing strokes and Alzheimer's disease, while reducing LDL cholesterol levels. Rosuvastatin, the newest statin drug, approved in August 2003, was shown in research trials to reduce LDL cholesterol levels by as much as 62 percent in as little as six weeks.

Angiotensin-Converting Enzyme (ACE) Inhibitors: These are medications that widen or dilate the blood vessels to improve the amount of blood the heart pumps and to lower blood pressure. ACE inhibitors also increase blood flow, which helps to decrease the amount of work your heart has to do. They belong to a class of drugs known as vasodilators. A persistent cough is the most common side effect of ACE inhibitors.

Angiotensin II Receptor Blockers (ARBs): These medications have the same effects as ACE inhibitors but work by a different mechanism. They decrease the action of certain chemicals that narrow the blood vessels, allowing blood to flow more easily. They also help to decrease certain chemicals that cause salt and fluid buildup.

Beta-blockers: These are medications that improve the heart's ability to relax and also decrease the production of harmful substances produced by the body in response to heart failure. Beta-blockers reduce heart rate and, over time, improve the heart's pumping ability.

Calcium Channel Blockers: These are medications designed to prevent the movement of calcium ions in the cells of the heart and blood vessels. As a result, calcium channel blockers relax blood vessels and increase the supply of blood and oxygen to the heart, while reducing its workload.

Aspirin: For over one hundred years, aspirin has been used as a pain reliever. Since the 1970s, aspirin has also been used to prevent and manage heart disease. Aspirin fights pain and inflammation associated with heart disease by blocking the action of an enzyme called cyclo-oxygenase. When this enzyme is blocked, the body is less able to produce a substance called prostaglandin, which is a chemical that signals an injury and "turns on" pain. Some of the prostaglandins in the blood trigger a series of events that cause blood platelets to clump together and form blood clots. By inhibiting prostaglandins, aspirin also inhibits the formation of blood clots.

Diuretics: Diuretics help the kidneys excrete unneeded water and salt through the urine. Ridding the system of excess fluid makes it easier for your heart to pump efficiently.

Procedures and Surgeries

Balloon Angioplasty: During this procedure, a specially designed catheter with a small balloon tip is guided to the point of narrowing in the artery. Once in place, the balloon is inflated to compress the plaque narrowing the arterial wall and stretch the artery open to increase blood flow to the heart. The possibility of complications—scarring, inflammation, and further blocking of the artery—is reduced if a stent (see below) is also implanted during the angioplasty.

Stent: A stent is a small stainless steel mesh tube that acts as a scaffold to provide support inside your coronary artery. A balloon catheter, placed over a guide wire, is used to insert the stent into the narrowed coronary artery. Once in place, the balloon tip is inflated, the stent is expanded to the size of the artery, and the artery is held open. The balloon is deflated and removed, and the stent is left permanently in place. Over a period of several weeks, the artery heals around the stent.

Newer stents are coated with an anti-inflammatory medication to prevent the overgrowth of scar tissue (and thus a further blockage and possible heart attack). Other stents are given a low dosage of radiation to
prevent overgrowth of scar tissue or a further blockage.

Coronary Bypass Surgery: When the coronary arteries are blocked,
new pathways to the heart may be needed. During coronary artery bypass graft surgery (also called CABG, or "cabbage"), a blood vessel is
removed or redirected from one area of the body—usually the leg—
and placed around the area of narrowing to "bypass" it and restore
blood flow to the heart muscle. This vessel is called a graft.

During traditional CABG, a surgeon makes an incision (about six
to eight inches) down the center of the sternum (breastbone) to get di-
rect access to the heart. The patient is connected to a heart-lung bypass machine, which allows for continuous circulation of blood
throughout the body during surgery. The heart is generally stopped for
thirty to ninety minutes of the surgery, which takes four or five hours.

After surgery, the surgeon closes the breastbone with special ster-
nal wires and the chest with special internal or traditional external
stitches.

During minimally invasive bypass surgery, the surgeon performs
the surgery through a small incision (about three inches) in the chest.
A common form of this surgery is called "off pump," or beating heart
surgery. This procedure allows surgeons to perform surgery while the
heart is still beating. The heart-lung machine is not used. The surgeon
uses advanced operating equipment to stabilize portions of the heart
and bypass the blocked artery. Meanwhile, the rest of the heart keeps
pumping and circulating blood to the body.

Robotic Bypass Surgery: The future is now. A robot assisting in the
operating room has become a fact, although not yet widely available.
The advantages are many. A robotic device can allow the operating surgeon greater dexterity while using a far less invasive procedure than
normal bypass surgery permits. Sophisticated cameras and tools can get
into the area of the body being operated on with modest half-inch or
smaller incisions, causing far less trauma to the patient. Even after un-
dergoing extensive heart surgery, many people are able to go home the

very next day. This is an extraordinary advance in bypass surgery, which, as it comes into greater use, offers both patients and physicians advantages unheard of until recently.

Nanotechnology: With robotic surgery still in its infancy, nanotechnology seems almost a gleam in a scientist's eye. However, research is ongoing, and in just the last couple of years, scientists have been able to create nanobots—tiny biologic mechanisms so minute that they can only be viewed through powerful microscopes. In the near future, nanobots will be utilized to perform a variety of diagnostic tests and repairs. These infinitesimal voyagers will be directed to muscles, organs, arteries, and veins throughout our systems to carry out any number of miraculously delicate tasks. We will have entered the future by then, and medical science will look back on our present as we now look back on our own medical history, marveling at how far science and technology have come in such a relatively short period of time.

Cardioversion: Cardioversion is a treatment for heart rhythms that are irregular—called arrhythmias. During cardioversion, a special machine is used to send electrical energy to the heart muscle to restore normal rhythm. The procedure restores the normal heart rate and rhythm, allowing the heart to pump more effectively. Cardioversion can be used to treat many types of fast and/or irregular heart rhythms. Most often, it is used to treat atrial fibrillation or atrial flutter. But cardioversion may also be used to treat ventricular tachycardia, another arrhythmia that can lead to a dangerous condition called ventricular fibrillation (a cause of sudden death.) The newest devices, the implantable cardioverter-defibrillator, is designed to perform dual functions—to act as a pacemaker to provide missing "beats" to a slowed heart rhythm and to send a fast, irregular heartbeat a powerful and precise electrical shock that keeps ventricular fibrillation from occurring. The normal, healthy heart has its own pacemaker that regulates the rate of heart beats.

Pacemaker: Often a pacemaker device can correct an irregular heartbeat. The pacemaker has two parts: the leads and a pulse generator. The pulse generator is implanted just under the skin of the chest, and the leads are threaded through the veins into the heart and implanted into the heart muscle. The electrical signals travel from the pulse generator to the leads. There are different types of pacemakers. Some have one lead, pacing only the ventricles or the atria; others have two leads, pacing both chambers. The single-chamber pacemaker has one lead in the upper or lower chamber of the heart. The dual-chamber pacemaker has one lead in the upper chamber and one lead in the lower chamber of the heart.

Implantable Cardioverter: Defibrillators combine the function of a pacemaker with the function of a cardioverter, protecting against abnormally low heartbeats (the pacemaker) and abnormally fast heartbeats (the cardioverter-defibrillator).

Fighting Cardiovascular Disease with the Blood Type Diet

The Blood Type Diet is designed to work in a complementary fashion with any of these treatments. I strongly recommend that before you begin this program, you sit down with your doctor and nutritionist and make sure you're all on the same page. Devise a schedule for checking your progress on the Blood Type Diet.

The cardiovascular blood type plan utilizes the best of naturopathic medicine, combined with individualized diet, exercise, and lifestyle strategies that support maximum health. The Blood Type Diet is nutritionally tailored to emphasize foods that support digestive, immune, and metabolic balance. The Blood Type Diet will help you lose weight and gain active tissue mass by including only the most efficiently digested and metabolized foods for your blood type. In most of my patients following the plan, there is a simultaneous reduction in LDL cholesterol and triglyceride levels.

If you are a heart surgery patient, the Blood Type Diet will help you more quickly regain strength and fitness and will become a powerful tool for avoiding a recurrence of your illness.

To summarize, your action plan to fight cardiovascular disease with the Blood Type Diet will include:

1. Minimizing foods that detract from proper metabolic function, create insulin resistance, and contribute to arterial damage.
2. Using the Blood Type Diet to minimize arterial inflammation and damage, while promoting repair and healing.
3. Engaging in blood type–specific exercise and lifestyle changes that reduce stress and further build lean muscle mass.
4. Controlling intake of harmful saturated fats, cholesterol, and trans-fatty acids.
5. Using specific supplements as a powerful adjunct to conventional treatment and prevention.

Are you ready to begin? Find your blood type–specific section, and we'll provide the right diet for your type to help in the fight against cardiovascular disease.

PART II

Individualized
Blood Type
Plans

Blood Type

O

BLOOD TYPE O DIET OUTCOME: SPECTACULAR RESULTS
"My results with the Blood Type Diet were quite spectacular. I was diagnosed as diabetic with high blood pressure, angina, and heart ischemia. I was following a diet prescribed by my cardiologist to the letter, along with medication, but the pain (pins and needles, numbness, headaches, joint pain, burning sensations) simply continued to get worse. Within two weeks of starting the Type O Diet, the pain had diminished and my general well-being had improved. I cut out most of my medication within two weeks and have been entirely free of it for about a month. My lab tests and blood pressure have all improved considerably."

BLOOD TYPE O DIET OUTCOME: THE NUMBERS TELL THE TALE
"In February, my cholesterol was 286, with triglycerides of 4. I started the Type O Diet at the beginning of March, and have been about 80 percent compliant. On June 4, my cholesterol was 214 and triglycerides were 2. I was very happy with these results."

Self-reported outcomes from the Blood Type Diet Web site (www.dadamo.com)

THE PATHWAY TO CARDIOVASCULAR DISEASE FOR BLOOD Type O is most likely to involve carbohydrate intolerance. As a modern Blood Type O, you retain the genetic imperative of your hunter-gatherer ancestors, giving you the ability to efficiently metabolize lean animal protein. However, a high-carbohydrate diet, containing metabolically inactivating lectins for Blood Type O, produces the type of weight gain associated with cardiovascular disease.

Blood Type O's cardiovascular health is dependent upon maintaining high active tissue mass and low body fat. A carbohydrate-dense diet produces the opposite state. The lectins in many grains and beans have insulin-mimicking effects on the insulin receptors of your fat cells. However, unlike insulin, which is cleaved off the receptor in about 30 minutes, these lectins remain permanently attached and continually signal your fat cells to stop burning fat and to store extra calories as fat. In effect, eating these lectins results in your body scavenging any extra carbohydrate sugars and converting them to unwanted fat. This

---

Blood Type O

TOP TWELVE HEART-HEALTHY FOODS

1. Lean, organic, grass-fed red meat
2. Richly oiled cold-water fish
3. Olive oil
4. Walnuts
5. Seaweeds
6. Broccoli
7. Spinach, kale, collards
8. Maitake mushrooms
9. Pineapple
10. Blueberries, cherries, elderberries
11. Turmeric
12. Green tea

syndrome also impairs triglyceride conversion and slows the production of thyroid hormone—factors in further weight gain and heart disease risk.

Eventually, carbohydrate intolerance produces insulin resistance, obesity, and high triglycerides—a combination classified as metabolic syndrome, a gateway to cardiovascular disease.

The Blood Type O Survival Factor

WHEN THE FAMOUS Framingham (Massachusetts) Heart Study examined the connection between blood type and heart disease, it analyzed rates of survival among different blood types. The study found that Blood Type O heart patients between the ages of thirty-nine and seventy-two had a much higher rate of survival than Blood Type A heart patients in the same age group. This was especially true for men between the ages of fifty and fifty-nine.

Although the study did not explore the subject in real depth, it appears that the same factors involved in Blood Type O's ability to survive heart disease also offer some protection against getting it in the first place. These factors include high levels of intestinal alkaline phosphatase and low levels of certain blood clotting factors.

As we discussed in chapter 2, intestinal alkaline phosphatase is an enzyme manufactured in the small intestine, which has the primary function of splitting dietary cholesterol and fats, aiding their efficient digestion and metabolism. Blood Type O has naturally high levels of this enzyme, and protein consumption increases the levels even further. As a result, Blood Type O can more easily digest animal protein and fat.

The second reason Blood Type O may enjoy better survival rates from heart disease is low levels of the blood clotting factors, factor VIII and von Willebrand Factor. As a result, Blood Type O has naturally "thinner" blood. This defect might actually work to Blood Type O's advantage when it comes to coronary artery disease, since thinner blood is less likely to deposit plaque that impedes arterial flow.

Finally, Blood Type O individuals tend to have higher levels of

digestive factors in the stomach, such as hydrochloric acid, pepsino-
gen, and gastrin. They don't suffer the cardiac consequences of a high-
protein diet as often as the other blood types because they metabolize
protein and fat much more efficiently.

Blood Type O: The Foods

THE BLOOD TYPE O Cardiovascular Diet is specifically adapted for
the prevention and management of cardiovascular disease. A new
category, **Super Beneficial,** highlights powerful disease-fighting foods
for Blood Type O. The **Neutral** category has also been adjusted to de-
emphasize foods that are less advantageous for you. Foods designated
Neutral: Allowed Infrequently should be minimized or avoided
entirely.

Food Values

SUPER BENEFICIAL	Foods that are known to have specific disease-fighting qualities for your blood type.
BENEFICIAL	Foods with components that enhance the metabolic, immune, or structural health of you blood type.
NEUTRAL: Allowed Infrequently	Foods that normally have no direct type effect but may impede your progress when consumed regularly.
AVOID	Foods with components that are harmful to your blood type.

Your secretor status can influence your ability to fully digest and metabolize certain foods, so various adjustments in the values are made for non-secretors. If you do not know your secretor type, the odds are that you can safely use the "secretor" values, since the majority of the population (approximately 80 percent) are secretors. However, I urge you to get tested, since the variations are important for non-secretors who want to maximize the effectiveness of the Blood Type Diet.

The food charts are divided into three sections. The top of the chart suggests the average portion size and quantity per week or day, according to secretor status. These recommendations do *not* apply to the category **Neutral: Allowed Infrequently**; those foods should be eaten rarely, if at all. The charts also indicate differences in frequency for some foods, based on ethnic heritage. It has been my experience that this factor has an impact upon the individual's ability to fully digest certain foods. For the purposes of blood type food choices, persons of Hispanic heritage should follow the recommendations for Caucasians; North American Native peoples should follow the recommendations for Asians.

The middle section of the chart gives the food values. The bottom section lists variants based on secretor status.

For your convenience, we have included a number of product names (Ezekiel 4:9 bread, Worcestershire sauce, etc.). However, keep in mind that commercial formulations vary among brands and regions. Even though a product may be listed as acceptable for you, always check its ingredients; do not use products that contain **Avoid** ingredients for your blood type. Of course, you may choose to make your own version of commercial products, such as bread and mayonnaise, using ingredients that suit your blood type. There are hundreds of delicious recipes for every blood type available on our Web site (www.dadamo.com) and in the book *Cook Right 4 Your Type: The Practical Kitchen Companion to* Eat Right 4 Your Type.

Meat/Poultry

A high-protein diet is the centerpiece of Blood Type O's heart-healthy strategy. Inadequate protein intake can seriously interfere with your

BLOOD TYPE O: MEAT/POULTRY			
Portion: 4–6 oz (men); 2–5 oz (women and children)			
	African	**Caucasian**	**Asian**
Secretor	6–9	6–9	6–9
Non-Secretor	7–12	7–12	7–11
		Times per week	

ability to metabolize fats, leading to a range of metabolic problems, including obesity, insulin resistance, diabetes, and heart disease. Choose only the best-quality (preferably grass-fed) chemical-, antibiotic-, and pesticide-free low-fat meats and poultry. Lean beef is a significant source of the amino acid carnitine (three ounces contain 81 mg). Carnitine is critical for the production of energy in heart muscle.

SUPER BENEFICIAL	BENEFICIAL	NEUTRAL: Allowed Frequently	NEUTRAL: Allowed Infrequently	AVOID
Beef	Heart (calf)	Chicken		All commercially processed meats
Buffalo	Sweet-	Cornish		
Lamb	breads	hen		
Liver (calf)	Venison	Duck		Bacon/Ham/ Pork
Mutton		Goat		Quail
Veal		Goose		Turtle
		Grouse		
		Guinea hen		
		Horse		
		Ostrich		
		Partridge		
		Pheasant		
		Rabbit		
		Squab		
		Squirrel		
		Turkey		

Special Variants: *Non-Secretor* BENEFICIAL: ostrich, partridge, pheasant, rabbit, squab; NEUTRAL (Allowed Frequently): lamb, liver (calf), quail, turtle.

Fish/Seafood

Fish and other seafoods represent a secondary source of high-quality protein for Blood Type O. In particular, richly oiled cold-water fish are high in omega-3 fatty acids, which can improve your metabolism and lower LDL (bad) cholesterol. Halibut is SUPER BENEFICIAL for cardio-conscious Blood Type Os. Three ounces has 40 mcg of the essential element selenium, which is increasingly considered critical to reducing arterial inflammation.

BLOOD TYPE O: FISH/SEAFOOD			
Portion: 4–6 oz (men); 2–5 oz (women and children)			
	African	Caucasian	Asian
Secretor	2–4	3–5	2–5
Non-Secretor	2–5	4–5	4–5
		Times per week	

SUPER BENEFICIAL	BENEFICIAL	NEUTRAL: Allowed Frequently	NEUTRAL: Allowed Infrequently	AVOID
Cod	Bass (all)	Anchovy	Eel	Abalone
Halibut	Perch (all)	Beluga	Flounder	Barracuda
Red snapper	Pike	Bluefish	Gray sole	Catfish
Trout (rainbow)	Shad	Bullhead	Grouper	Conch
	Sole (except gray)	Butterfish	Whitefish	Frog
	Sturgeon	Carp		Herring (pickled/ smoked)
	Swordfish	Caviar (sturgeon)		Muskellunge
	Tilefish	Chub		Octopus
	Yellowtail	Clam		Pollock
		Crab		Salmon roe
		Croaker		Salmon (smoked)
		Cusk		
		Drum		
		Haddock		

SUPER BENEFICIAL	BENEFICIAL	NEUTRAL: Allowed Frequently	NEUTRAL: Allowed Infrequently	AVOID
		Hake		Squid (calamari)
		Halfmoon fish		
		Harvest fish		
		Herring (fresh)		
		Lobster		
		Mackerel		
		Mahi-mahi		
		Monkfish		
		Mullet		
		Mussel		
		Opaleye		
		Orange roughy		
		Oyster		
		Parrot fish		
		Pickerel		
		Pompano		
		Porgy		
		Rosefish		
		Sailfish		
		Salmon		
		Sardine		
		Scallop		
		Scrod		
		Shark		
		Shrimp		
		Smelt		
		Snail (*Helix pomatia/* escargot)		

SUPER BENEFICIAL	BENEFICIAL	NEUTRAL: Allowed Frequently	NEUTRAL: Allowed Infrequently	AVOID
		Sucker		
		Sunfish		
		Tilapia		
		Trout (brook/ sea)		
		Tuna		
		Weakfish		
		Whiting		

Special Variants: *Non-Secretor* BENEFICIAL: hake, herring (fresh), mackerel, sardine; NEUTRAL (Allowed Frequently): bass, catfish, halibut, salmon roe, red snapper; AVOID: anchovy, crab, mussel.

Dairy/Eggs

Most dairy foods should be avoided by Blood Type O. They are poorly digested and metabolized. In the absence of dairy foods, a daily calcium supplement is advised, especially for postmenopausal Type O women.

Ghee (clarified butter) is one exception because it's a good source of butyrate, which supports Blood Type O intestinal health. Eggs can be consumed in moderation. They are a good source of docosahexaenoic acid (DHA) and can help you build active tissue mass. Do your best to find eggs and dairy products that meet organic standards.

BLOOD TYPE O: EGGS			
Portion: 1 egg			
	African	Caucasian	Asian
Secretor	1–4	3–6	3–4
Non-Secretor	2–5	3–6	3–4
		Times per week	

BLOOD TYPE O: MILK AND YOGURT			
Portion: 4–6 oz (men); 2–5 oz (women and children)			
	African	Caucasian	Asian
Secretor	0–1	0–3	0–2
Non-Secretor	0	0–2	0–3
		Times per week	

BLOOD TYPE O: CHEESE			
Portion: 3 oz (men); 2 oz (women and children)			
	African	Caucasian	Asian
Secretor	0–1	0–2	0–1
Non-Secretor	0	0–1	0
		Times per week	

SUPER BENEFICIAL	BENEFICIAL	NEUTRAL: Allowed Frequently	NEUTRAL: Allowed Infrequently	AVOID
	Ghee (clarified butter)	Egg (chicken/ duck)	Butter Farmer cheese Feta Goat cheese Mozzarella	American cheese Blue cheese Brie Buttermilk Camembert Casein Cheddar Colby Cottage cheese Cream cheese Edam Egg (goose/ quail)

SUPER BENEFICIAL	BENEFICIAL	NEUTRAL: Allowed Frequently	NEUTRAL: Allowed Infrequently	AVOID
				Emmenthal
				Gouda
				Gruyère
				Half-and-half
				Ice cream
				Jarlsberg
				Kefir
				Milk (cow/goat)
				Monterey Jack
				Muenster
				Neufchâtel
				Paneer
				Parmesan
				Provolone
				Quark
				Ricotta
				Sherbet
				Sour cream
				String cheese
				Swiss cheese
				Whey
				Yogurt

Special Variants: *Non-Secretor* NEUTRAL (Allowed Frequently): Egg(goose/quail); AVOID: farmer cheese, feta, goat cheese, mozzarella.

Oils

Olive oil, a monounsaturated oil, is SUPER BENEFICIAL for Blood Type O. Constituents in olive oil, such as flavonoids, squalenes, and polyphenols, act as powerful antioxidants and may help lower bad (LDL) cholesterol. Use it as your primary cooking oil. Also SUPER BENEFICIAL is flax oil, high in alpha-linolenic acid, which has anti-inflammatory properties. Be aware that some oils are high in omega-6 fatty acids, which can stimulate arterial inflammation. These include corn, cottonseed, peanut, and safflower oils. Secretors have a bit of an edge over non-secretors in digesting oils and probably benefit a bit more from their consumption.

BLOOD TYPE O: OILS			
Portion: 1 tblsp			
	African	Caucasian	Asian
Secretor	3–8	4–8	5–8
Non-Secretor	1–7	3–5	3–6
		Times per week	

SUPER BENEFICIAL	BENEFICIAL	NEUTRAL: Allowed Frequently	NEUTRAL: Allowed Infrequently	AVOID
Flax (linseed) Olive		Almond Black currant seed Borage seed Cod liver Sesame Walnut	Canola	Avocado Castor Coconut Corn Cottonseed Evening primrose Peanut Safflower Soy Sunflower Wheat germ

Special Variants: *Non-Secretor* BENEFICIAL: almond, walnut; NEUTRAL (Allowed Frequently): coconut, flax; AVOID: borage, canola, cod liver.

Nuts and Seeds

Nuts and seeds are a secondary source of protein for Blood Type O. Walnuts are highly recommended, as they are known to be helpful in lowering cholesterol and triglycerides and regulating blood sugar. Flax (linseed) is an excellent source of fiber and can also help lower blood pressure, protect the arteries, and reduce the risk of heart attacks and strokes. Overall, however, your intake of vegetable protein sources such as nuts, seeds, and beans should be limited to the portions and frequencies recommended, because they do not build active tissue mass (calorie-burning cells) as efficiently as lean meats, fowl, and fish.

BLOOD TYPE O: NUTS AND SEEDS			
Portion: Whole (handful); Nut Butters (2 tblsp)			
	African	Caucasian	Asian
Secretor	2–5	2–5	2–4
Non-Secretor	5–7	5–7	5–7
			Times per week

SUPER BENEFICIAL	BENEFICIAL	NEUTRAL: Allowed Frequently	NEUTRAL: Allowed Infrequently	AVOID
Flax (linseed)	Pumpkin seed	Almond	Safflower seed	Beechnut
Walnut (black/English)		Almond butter	Sesame butter (tahini)	Brazil nut
		Almond cheese	Sesame seed	Cashew
		Almond milk		Chestnut
		Butternut		Litchi
		Filbert (hazelnut)		Peanut
		Hickory		Peanut butter
		Macadamia		Pistachio
		Pecan		Poppy seed
				Sunflower butter
				Sunflower seed

SUPER BENEFICIAL	BENEFICIAL	NEUTRAL: Allowed Frequently	NEUTRAL: Allowed Infrequently	AVOID
		Pignolia (pine nut)		

Special Variants: *Non-Secretor* NEUTRAL (Allowed Frequently): flax (linseed); AVOID: almond cheese, almond milk, safflower seed.

Beans and Legumes

Essentially a carnivore when it comes to protein requirements, Blood Type O can benefit from proteins found in some beans and legumes, although several of them contain problematic lectins. Given the choice, get your protein from animal foods.

Soy products are allowed for Blood Type O. If you've been accustomed to having dairy foods in your diet, soy milk and cheese can be substituted occasionally.

BLOOD TYPE O: BEANS AND LEGUMES			
Portion: 1 cup (cooked)			
	African	Caucasian	Asian
Secretor	1–3	1–3	2–4
Non-Secretor	0–2	0–3	2–4
		Times per week	

SUPER BENEFICIAL	BENEFICIAL	NEUTRAL: Allowed Frequently	NEUTRAL: Allowed Infrequently	AVOID
Bean (green/ snap/ string) Fava (broad) bean	Adzuki bean Black-eyed pea	Black bean Cannellini bean Garbanzo (chick- pea) Jicama bean	Soy milk	Copper bean Kidney bean Lentil (all) Navy bean Pinto bean Tamarind bean

SUPER BENEFICIAL	BENEFICIAL	NEUTRAL: Allowed Frequently	NEUTRAL: Allowed Infrequently	AVOID
Northern bean		Lima bean	Soy milk	
		Miso		
		Mung bean/ sprouts		
		Pea (green/ pod/ snow)		
		Soy bean		
		Soy cheese		
		Tempeh		
		Tofu		
		White bean		

Special Variants: *Non-Secretor* NEUTRAL (Allowed Frequently): adzuki bean, black-eyed pea, lentil (all), pinto bean. AVOID: fava (broad) bean, garbanzo (chickpea), soy (all).

Grains and Starches

Grains and starches are the Achilles' heel of Blood Type O. You tend to do poorly on corn, wheat, sorghum, barley, and many of their by-products (sweeteners, etc.). These common grains have a very pronounced effect on increasing body fat, raising triglycerides, and promoting insulin resistance—thus increasing the risk of cardiovascular disease for Blood Type O. The exceptions are sprouted seed breads, such as Essene and Ezekiel, usually found in the freezer section of your health-food store. The gluten lectins, principally found in the seed coats, are destroyed in the sprouting process. Unlike many commercially sprouted breads, Essene and Ezekiel are "live" foods, with many beneficial enzymes intact.

BLOOD TYPE O: GRAINS AND STARCHES

Portion: ½ cup dry (grains or pastas); 1 muffin; 2 slices of bread

	African	Caucasian	Asian
Secretor	1–6	1–6	1–6
Non-Secretor	0–3	0–3	0–3
		Times per week	

SUPER BENEFICIAL	BENEFICIAL	NEUTRAL: Allowed Frequently	NEUTRAL: Allowed Infrequently	AVOID
	Essene bread (manna)	Amaranth	Buckwheat	Barley
		Ezekiel 4:9 bread	Millet	Cornmeal
		Kamut	Oat bran	Couscous
		Quinoa	Oat flour	Grits
		Spelt (whole)	Oatmeal	Popcorn
		Spelt flour/ products	Rice (whole)	Sorghum
		Tapioca	Rice (wild)	Wheat (refined/ un-bleached)
		Teff	Rice cake	Wheat (semolina)
		100% sprouted grain products (except Essene)	Rice flour	Wheat (white flour)
			Rice milk	Wheat (whole)
			Rye (whole)	Wheat bran
			Rye flour/ products	Wheat germ
			Soba noodles (100% buck-wheat)	
			Soy flour/ products	

Special Variants: *Non-Secretor* AVOID: buckwheat, oat (all), soba noodles (100% buckwheat), soy flour/products, spelt (whole), spelt flour/products, tapioca.

Vegetables

Vegetables provide a treasure trove of antioxidants and fiber, and several—especially mushrooms, broccoli, and greens—support cardiovascular health. Leafy green vegetables, such as kale, collards, broccoli, and spinach, are rich sources of the blood clotting vitamin K, necessary for Type O with your "thin" blood. Seaweeds help Blood Type O regulate thyroid function. Maitake mushrooms can help regulate metabolism. Many vegetables recommended for Blood Type O are also rich in potassium, which helps lower extracellular water in the body—a source of edema.

Certain vegetables from the Brassica family, such as cauliflower and mustard greens, can inhibit thyroid function and should be avoided. Cabbage should be avoided by non-secretors and limited by secretors. Alfalfa sprouts can also inhibit thyroid activity for Blood Type O.

An item's value also applies to its juice, unless otherwise noted.

BLOOD TYPE O: VEGETABLES			
Portion: 1 cup, prepared (cooked or raw)			
	African	Caucasian	Asian
Secretor Super/ Beneficials	Unlimited	Unlimited	Unlimited
Secretor Neutrals	2–5	2–5	2–5
Non-Secretor Super/ Beneficials	Unlimited	Unlimited	Unlimited
Non-Secretor Neutrals	2–3	2–3	2–3
			Times per day

SUPER BENEFICIAL	BENEFICIAL	NEUTRAL: Allowed Frequently	NEUTRAL: Allowed Infrequently	AVOID
Beet greens	Artichoke	Arugula	Brussels sprouts	Alfalfa sprouts
Broccoli	Dandelion	Asparagus	Cabbage	Aloe
Chicory	Horse-radish	Asparagus pea		Cauliflower

SUPER BENEFICIAL	BENEFICIAL	NEUTRAL: Allowed Frequently	NEUTRAL: Allowed Infrequently	AVOID
Collards	Kohlrabi	Bamboo shoot	Olive (Greek/ green/ Spanish)	Corn
Escarole	Lettuce (Romaine)	Beet		Cucumber
Kale		Bok choy	Yam	Leek
Mushroom (maitake)	Mushroom (abalone/ enoki/ oyster/ porto- bello/ straw/ tree ear)	Carrot		Mushroom (shiitake/ silver dollar)
Seaweeds		Celeriac		Mustard greens
Spinach		Celery		Olive (black)
Swiss Chard		Chili pepper		Potato
	Okra	Daikon radish		
	Onion (all)	Eggplant		
	Parsnip	Endive		
	Potato (sweet)	Fennel		
	Pumpkin	Fiddlehead fern		
	Turnip	Garlic		
		Lettuce (except Romaine)		
		Peppers (all)		
		Poi		
		Radicchio		
		Radish/ sprouts		
		Rappini (broccoli rabe)		
		Rutabaga		
		Scallion		
		Shallot		
		Squash		

SUPER BENEFICIAL	BENEFICIAL	NEUTRAL: Allowed Frequently	NEUTRAL: Allowed Infrequently	AVOID
		Tomato		
		Water chestnut		
		Watercress		
		Zucchini		

Special Variants: *Non-Secretor* BENEFICIAL: carrot, fiddlehead fern, garlic; NEU-TRAL (Allowed Frequently): lettuce (Romaine), mushroom (except shiitake), parsn potato (sweet), turnip; NEUTRAL (Allowed Infrequently): mustard greens; AVOID: Brussels sprouts, cabbage, eggplant, olive (all), poi.

Fruits and Fruit Juices

Eating plenty of fruit favorable to Blood Type O can improve yo overall metabolic function and help you maintain a healthy weig. Many, such as blueberries, cherries, and elderberries, contain polysac charides that encourage weight loss by tempering the effects of insulin. Also, fruits can help shift the balance of water in the body from high extracellular concentrations to high intracellular concentrations. Man fruits, such as pineapple, are rich in enzymes that can help reduce in flammation and prevent water retention.

Grapefruit juice is a well-documented culprit in many food-dru interactions. Grapefruit juice can inhibit the metabolism of certa heart and blood pressure drugs, including Nifedipine, Verapamil, a Lovastatin. Many readers have reported cautionary warnings of grap fruit's interaction appearing on Coumadin (warfarin prescriptio blood thinners). There is no evidence in the medical literature to s port this interaction. Grapefruit's effect on warfarin is insignific

An item's value also applies to its juices, unless otherwise no

BLOOD TYPE O: FR UITS AND FRUIT JUICES			
Portion: 1 cup			
	African	Caucasian	Asian
Secretor	2–4	3–5	3–5
Non-Secretor	1–3	1–3	1–3
	Times per day		

SUPER BENEFICIAL	BENEFICIAL	NEUTRAL: Allowed Frequently	NEUTRAL: Allowed Infrequently	AVOID
Blueberry	Banana	Boysen- berry	Apple	Asian pear
Cherry	Fig (fresh/ dried)	Breadfruit	Apricot	Avocado
Elderberry (dark blue/ purple)	Guava	Canang melon	Currant	Bitter melon
Pineapple	Mango	Casaba melon	Date	Blackberry
Plum		Christmas melon	Grapes (all)	Cantaloupe
Prune		Cranberry	Quince	Coconut
		Crenshaw melon	Raisin	Honeydew
		Dewberry	Star fruit (caram- bola)	Kiwi
		Gooseberry	Strawberry	Orange
		Grapefruit		Plantain
		Kumquat		Tangerine
		Lemon		
		Lime		
		Loganberry		
		Mulberry		
		Musk- melon		
		Nectarine		
		Papaya		
		Peach		
		Pear		

SUPER BENEFICIAL	BENEFICIAL	NEUTRAL: Allowed Frequently	NEUTRAL: Allowed Infrequently	AVOID
		Persian melon		
		Persimmon		
		Pomegranate		
		Prickly pear		
		Raspberry		
		Sago palm		
		Spanish melon		
		Watermelon		
		Youngberry		

Special Variants: *Non-Secretor:* BENEFICIAL: avocado, pomegranate, prickly pear; NEUTRAL (Allowed Frequently): elderberry (dark blue/purple); AVOID: apple, apricot, date, strawberry.

Spices/Condiments/Sweeteners

Many spices have mild to moderate medicinal properties, often through their influence upon the balance of bacteria in the lower intestine, enabling the proper digestion and metabolism of foods. For Blood Type O, fenugreek is SUPER BENEFICIAL for its cardiovascular effects, which include lowering triglycerides. Turmeric is also SUPER BENEFICIAL because of a powerful chemical called curcumin, which helps improve liver function.

Many common food additives, such as guar gum and carrageenan, should be avoided as they can enhance the effects of lectins found in other foods. Use caution when using prepared condiments, as they often contain wheat.

SUPER BENEFICIAL	BENEFICIAL	NEUTRAL: Allowed Frequently	NEUTRAL: Allowed Infrequently	AVOID
Fenugreek	Carob	Agar	Apple	Aspartame
Turmeric	Ginger	Allspice	pectin	Caper
	Horse-	Almond	Arrowroot	Carrageenan
	radish	extract	Barley	Cornstarch
	Parsley	Anise	malt	Corn syrup
	Pepper	Basil	Chocolate	Dextrose
	(cayenne)	Bay leaf	Honey	Fructose
		Bergamot	Ketchup	Guarana
		Caraway	Maple	Gums (aca-
		Cardamom	syrup	cia/Ara-
		Chervil	Molasses	bic/guar)
		Chili	Molasses	Invert sugar
		powder	(black-	Juniper
		Chive	strap)	Mace
		Cilantro	Rice syrup	Malto-
		(corian-	Senna	dextrin
		der leaf)	Soy sauce	MSG
		Cinnamon	Sucanat	Nutmeg
		Clove	Sugar	Pepper
		Coriander	(brown/	(black/
		Cream of	white)	white)
		tartar		Vinegar (ex-
		Cumin		cept apple
		Dill		cider)
		Garlic		Worcester-
		Gelatin,		shire sauce
		plain		
		Lecithin		
		Licorice		
		root*		
		Marjoram		

SUPER BENEFICIAL	BENEFICIAL	NEUTRAL: Allowed Frequently	NEUTRAL: Allowed Infrequently	AVOID
		Mayonnaise		
		Mint (all)		
		Mustard (dry)		
		Oregano		
		Paprika		
		Pepper (peppercorn/red flakes)		
		Rosemary		
		Saffron		
		Sage		
		Savory		
		Sea salt		
		Stevia		
		Tamari (wheat-free)		
		Tamarind		
		Tarragon		
		Thyme		
		Vanilla		
		Vegetable glycerine		
		Vinegar (apple cider)		
		Wintergreen		

SUPER BENEFICIAL	BENEFICIAL	NEUTRAL: Allowed Frequently	NEUTRAL: Allowed Infrequently	AVOID
		Yeast (baker's/ brewer's)		

Special Variants: *Non-Secretor* BENEFICIAL: basil, bay leaf, licorice root*, oregano, saffron, tarragon, yeast (brewer's); NEUTRAL (Allowed Frequently): carob, MSG, turmeric; AVOID: agar, barley malt, cinnamon, honey, maple syrup, mayonnaise, rice syrup, sage, soy sauce, stevia, sucanat, sugar (brown/white), tamari (wheat-free), vanilla, vinegar (apple cider).

*Do not use if you have high blood pressure.

Herbal Teas

Herbal teas can provide medicinal benefits and are excellent replacements for caffeinated drinks such as coffee, cola, and black tea. In particular, dandelion supports Blood Type O metabolism, and fenugreek can directly influence cardiovascular function.

SUPER BENEFICIAL	BENEFICIAL	NEUTRAL: Allowed Frequently	NEUTRAL: Allowed Infrequently	AVOID
Dandelion	Chickweed	Catnip	Senna	Alfalfa
Fenugreek	Ginger	Chamomile		Aloe
	Hops	Dong quai		Burdock
	Linden	Elder		Coltsfoot
	Mulberry	Ginseng		Corn silk
	Peppermint	Hawthorn		Echinacea
	Rosehip	Horehound		Gentian
	Sarsaparilla	Licorice		Goldenseal
	Slippery elm	Mullein		Red clover
		Raspberry leaf		Rhubarb
		Skullcap		Shepherd's purse

SUPER BENEFICIAL	BENEFICIAL	NEUTRAL: Allowed Frequently	NEUTRAL: Allowed Infrequently	AVOID
		Spearmint Valerian Vervain White birch White oak bark Yarrow		St. John's wort Strawberry leaf Yellow dock
Special Variants: None.				

Miscellaneous Beverages

With the exception of red wine, avoid or limit alcohol, which can promote insulin resistance. Coffee can trigger a hypoglycemia-like reaction.

SUPER BENEFICIAL	BENEFICIAL	NEUTRAL: Allowed Frequently	NEUTRAL: Allowed Infrequently	AVOID
Tea (green)	Seltzer Soda (club)	Wine (red)		Beer Coffee (reg/ decaf) Liquor Soda (cola/diet/ misc.) Tea, black (reg/ decaf) Wine (white)
Special Variants: *Non-Secretor* BENEFICIAL: Wine (red).				

Supplements

THE BLOOD TYPE O Diet offers abundant quantities of important nutrients, such as protein and iron. It is important to get as many nutrients as possible from fresh foods and use supplements only to fill in the minor deficiencies in your diet. The following supplement protocols are designed for Blood Type O individuals who are suffering from cardiovascular disease or related conditions.

Note: If you are being treated for a cardiovascular or related condition, consult your doctor before taking any supplements.

Blood Type O: Cardiovascular Protection and Enhancement Protocol

Use this protocol for 4–8 weeks, then discontinue for 2 weeks and restart.		
SUPPLEMENT	**ACTION**	**DOSAGE**
L-carnitine	Enhances intracellular energy production; reduces blood pressure	500 mg, twice daily
Turmeric	Shows promise in lowering cholesterol levels and fighting atherosclerosis, a buildup of fatty deposits in the arteries	300–350 mg (containing 95% curcumin) twice day
Selenium	Helps reduce or prevent arterial inflammation	50 mcg daily

Blood Type O: Specific Cardiovascular Treatment Protocols

Use these protocols for 4–8 weeks, then discontinue for 1 week and restart. Protocols can be combined.		
Elevated Triglyceride, Cholesterol, or LDL Control*		
SUPPLEMENT	**ACTION**	**DOSAGE**
Green tea	High concentration of strong anti-oxidants called catechins increase the liver's LDL receptors.	2–4 cups daily
Guggul gum (*Commiphora mukul*)	Provides vascular support; lowers triglycerides	Standardized for 25 mg guggulsterones of type E and Z. 1 capsule, 1–2 times daily
Niacin (physician supervised)*	Helps decrease total cholesterol and LDL, and helps increase HDL. Niacin can cause flushing of the skin primarily on the face, arms, and chest, and may occur initially at doses as low as 30 mg/day. If you plan on using this part of the protocol, consult your physician.	50 mg daily
Stress Reduction Protocol		
SUPPLEMENT	**ACTION**	**DOSAGE**
Russian Rhodiola (*Rhodiola rosea*)	Prevents stress-induced cate-cholamine activity in the heart.	250 mg, three times daily

SUPPLEMENT	ACTION	DOSAGE
L-theanine	Anti-anxiety remedy	100–200 mg, twice daily
L-tyrosine*	Improves metabolic and thyroid function	500 mg, daily

Angina Relief Adjunct*		
SUPPLEMENT	**ACTION**	**DOSAGE**
Arjuna myrobalan (*Terminalia arjuna*) 2% arjunolic acid	Promotes cardiac health; used by Ayurvedic physicians to treat heart diseases such as endocarditis, mitral regurgitation, peri- carditis, and angina	250 mg, twice daily
Coenzyme Q-10	Increases intracellular energy; protects against angina	30 mg, twice daily with meals
Copper	May play a role in staving off heart rhythm disorders (arrhythmias) and high blood pressure	2 mg every other day. Should be combined with 15–25 mg of zinc

Hypertension Control*		
SUPPLEMENT	**ACTION**	**DOSAGE**
Dandelion (*Taraxacum officinale*)	Mild diuretic, rich in electrolytes	150 mg, twice daily
Coleus (*Coleus forskohlii*)	Enhances intracellular energy production; reduces blood pressure	Standardized extract, 125 mg, once daily
Magnesium	Mild to moderate effects on blood pressure	500 mg, twice daily

Metabolic Control*		
SUPPLEMENT	**ACTION**	**DOSAGE**
Lipoic acid	Enhances insulin sensitivity	100 mg, twice daily
Bladderwrack (*Fucus vesiculosus*)	Improves metabolic function; regulates thyroid activity	200 mg, daily
N-acetyl glucosamine (NAG)	Blocks anti-metabolic lectins in grains and other Blood Type O AVOIDS	300–600 mg taken with large meals

*Check with your doctor before beginning this or any other nutritional protocol, especially if you are currently taking prescription medication.

The Exercise Component

EXERCISE IS KEY to cardiovascular health, and this is especially true for Blood Type O. You benefit tremendously from brisk regular exercise that taxes your cardiovascular and musculoskeletal systems. Your goal should be to develop as much active tissue mass as possible; this is the key to your metabolic fitness.

Exercise is also crucial to a well-regulated chemical release system. The act of physical exercise releases a swarm of neurotransmitter activity that acts as a tonic for the entire system. More than any other blood type, Blood Type O requires regular, high-intensity exercise to maintain physical health and emotional balance. Below is a list of exercises that are recommended for Blood Type O, along with some general tips for making the most of your exercise program. Build a balanced routine of both aerobic and strength-training activities from the following options:

EXERCISE	DURATION	FREQUENCY
Aerobics	40–60 minutes	3–4 x week
Weight training	30–45 minutes	3–4 x week
Running	40–45 minutes	3–4 x week
Calisthenics	30–45 minutes	3 x week
Treadmill	30 minutes	3 x week
Kickboxing	30–45 minutes	3 x week
Cycling	30 minutes	3 x week
Contact sports	60 minutes	2–3 x week
In-line/roller skating	30 minutes	2–3 x week

3 Steps to Effective Exercise

1. Warm up with stretching and flexibility moves before you start your aerobic exercise.
2. To achieve maximum cardiovascular benefits, work toward an elevated heart rate that is about 70 percent of your capacity. Once you reach the elevated rate, continue exercising to maintain that rate for twenty to thirty minutes. To calculate your maximum heart rate and performance level:
   - Subtract your age from 220.
   - Multiply the difference by .70 (or .60 if you are over age sixty). This is the high end of your performance.
   - Multiply the remainder by .50. This is the low end of your performance.
3. Finish each aerobic session with at least a five-minute cooldown of stretching and relaxation moves.

Getting Started: The First Month

IF YOU ARE NEW to the Blood Type Diet, the following guidelines will introduce you to the Blood Type O regimen over a period of one month. Follow these recommendations as closely as possible, using a journal to record your personal experiences with the diet. In addition

Blood Type O Cardiovascular Diet Checklist

Eat small to moderate portions of high-quality, lean, organic ☐ meat several times a week for strength, energy, and digestive health. Meat should be prepared medium to rare for the best health effects. If you charbroil or cook meat well-done, use a marinade composed of beneficial ingredients, such as cherry juice, spices, and herbs.

Include regular portions of richly oiled cold-water fish. Fish ☐ oils can improve cardiac health, contribute to lower cholesterol and triglyceride levels, and support thyroid function.

Consume little or no dairy foods, as Blood Type O poorly di- ☐ gests them.

Eliminate wheat and wheat-based products from your diet. ☐ They are the gateway to metabolic syndrome and cardiovascular disease for your blood type.

Limit your intake of beans, as they are not a particularly good ☐ protein source for Type Os. Some contain reactive lectins that can impair metabolic activity.

Eat lots of BENEFICIAL fruits and vegetables. ☐

If you need a daily dose of caffeine, replace coffee with green ☐ tea. It isn't acidic and has substantially less caffeine than a cup of coffee.

Use BENEFICIAL and NEUTRAL nuts and dried fruits for ☐ snacks.

to factors that are measurable in medical tests (i.e., EKGs, cholesterol levels, blood pressure, and cardiac stress tests), take the time to note changes in your energy levels, sleep patterns, digestion, and overall well-being.

Week 1

Blood Type Diet and Supplements

- Eliminate your most harmful AVOID foods—wheat and dairy. These foods interfere with Blood Type O's cardiovascular health.

- Include your most important BENEFICIAL foods on a regular schedule throughout the week. For example, have lean red meat 5 times and omega-3–rich fish 3 to 4 times, with lots of beneficial vegetables and fruit.

- Incorporate at least 1 SUPER BENEFICIAL food into your daily diet. For example, eat slices of fresh pineapple or a seaweed salad.

- If you're a coffee drinker, begin to wean yourself by cutting your daily consumption in half. I recommend substituting green tea, which has many SUPER BENEFICIAL qualities and delivers a small amount of caffeine.

Exercise Regimen

- Plan to exercise at least 4 days this week, for 45 minutes each day.

  2 days: aerobic activity

  2 days: weights

- If you experience angina during exercise, consult with a physician. Angina is a warning sign that some of your heart muscle is not getting enough oxygen.

- If you are not accustomed to aerobic exercise, start slowly, and gradually increase your duration and intensity of activity. The important factor is consistency. Just do it—as much as you're able.

- Use your journal to detail the time, activity, distance, and amount of weight. Note the number of repetitions for each exercise.

■ WEEK 1 SUCCESS STRATEGY ■
Make Time for Exercise

It's a common complaint: "My job is too demanding to fit exercise into my schedule." With a little creativity, you can incorporate physical activity into your regular routine. Here are some tips:

- If you hold daily or weekly staff meetings, skip the conference room and do your talking while walking.
- Take the stairs instead of the elevator.
- If your flight is delayed, walk around the airport instead of sitting at the food court.

- Stay at hotels with fitness centers and use them instead of the cocktail hour to relieve stress.
- Start a fitness club at your company and offer rewards, such as a day off, a bonus, or a gift certificate for employees who meet their goals.
- Get involved in an industry baseball, basketball, or soccer league.
- If you drive to work, park a mile from the office and walk the rest of the way. Or get off the bus or train at an earlier stop.

Week 2

Blood Type Diet and Supplements

- Begin to eliminate the next level of AVOID foods—corn, potatoes, beans, and legumes.
- Eat at least 2 BENEFICIAL animal proteins every day, choosing from the meat, poultry, and seafood lists.
- Initially, it is best to avoid foods listed as NEUTRAL: Allowed Infrequently.
- Continue to incorporate SUPER BENEFICIAL foods into your daily diet.
- If you're a coffee drinker, continue to cut your coffee intake, replacing it with BENEFICIAL herbal teas. Drink a cup of green tea every morning.

Exercise Regimen

- Continue to exercise at least 4 days this week, for 45 minutes each day.

  2 days: aerobic activity

  2 days: weights

■ WEEK 2 SUCCESS STRATEGY ■
Fight Carbohydrate Cravings

If you crave any form of stimulants or carbohydrates, your serotonin levels are low and your brain is demanding stimulants to raise your serotonin levels. Try drinking some unsweetened cocoa powder in hot water or in a protein smoothie. Chocolate contains small amounts of serotonin, which explains why we feel so good when we eat it. Try a sip of vegetable glycerine between meals to cut down on your cravings. Avoid using the herbal serotonin supplements (e.g., 5HTP) on the market. The source material (griffonia seed) has a Type O reactive lectin, which could be a problem.

Week 3

Blood Type Diet and Supplements

- When you plan your meals for week 3, choose BENEFICIAL or SUPER BENEFICIAL foods to replace NEUTRAL foods whenever possible. For example, choose lean, organic beef or buffalo over chicken, or blueberries over an apple.
- Eliminate all remaining AVOID foods.
- Liberally incorporate SUPER BENEFICIAL foods into your daily diet.
- Completely wean yourself from coffee, substituting green tea 2 to 3 times a day, as well as SUPER BENEFICIAL herbal teas.

Exercise Regimen

- Continue to exercise at least 4 days this week, for 45 minutes each day.

  2 days: aerobic activity

  2 days: weights

■ WEEK 3 SUCCESS STRATEGY ■
Heart-Healthy Alternatives

There's no need to feel deprived on the Blood Type Diet. Satisfy your cravings with these alternatives:

INSTEAD OF...		EAT...
processed sweets	→ → →	pineapple slices or raisins
salty foods	→ → →	nori (seaweed) or celery sticks
ice cream	→ → →	frozen fruit ice or sorbet
fatty foods	→ → →	a banana or walnuts
creamy foods	→ → →	vegetable puree, with 1 tblsp egg lecithin and 1 tblsp olive oil

Week 4

Blood Type Diet and Supplements

- Continue at the week 3 level, focusing on BENEFICIAL and SUPER BENEFICIAL foods.

- Evaluate the first 4 weeks and make adjustments.

Exercise Regimen

- Continue at the week 3 level.

- Review your progress, noting in your journal improvements in strength and flexibility. Determine which exercise regimen has worked for you, including time of day, setting, and activity level.

▪ WEEK 4 SUCCESS STRATEGY ▪
Watch the Belly Fat

Excess weight is most unhealthy—and most conducive to metabolic problems—when it is centered in your abdomen, as opposed to your hips and thighs. Here's a quick test to learn about your fat distribution: Stand straight in front of a full-length mirror. Using a tape measure, measure the distance around the smallest part of your waist. Now measure the distance around the largest part of your buttocks. Divide your waist measurement by your hip measurement. A healthy ratio for women is .70 to .75. A healthy ratio for men is .80 to .90.

A Final Word

IN SUMMARY, the secret to fighting cardiovascular disease with the Blood Type O Diet involves:

1. Increasing active tissue mass (calorie-burning tissue) by switching to a more protein–based diet.
2. Minimizing consumption of the insulin-mimicking lectins most abundant in grains such as wheat and corn, which can contribute to metabolic syndrome, a precursor to heart disease.
3. Increasing circulatory efficiency, lowering adrenaline, and minimizing arterial damage by adopting a vigorous exercise program.
4. Using supplements intelligently to block the effect of insulin-mimicking lectins, provide antioxidant support, and control triglyceride levels.

Blood Type

A

BLOOD TYPE A DIET OUTCOME: A REFORMED SKEPTIC

"My LDL cholesterol has been over 250 for years. No diet that I tried reduced it. In fact, the diets recommended by the doctors and nurses raised it. After a few short months on the Blood Type Diet, my LDL cholesterol had lowered over 100 points. I am going back to my doctor for another test, because he was skeptical. I'm *not* skeptical, because I know!"

BLOOD TYPE A DIET OUTCOME: NEW AND IMPROVED

"On September 20, 1999, I started the Blood Type Diet. I gave up wheat, dairy, red meat, sugar, and alcohol. I also stopped taking three of my doctor-prescribed meds (hormone, cholesterol, antidepressant). I began receiving acupuncture to help me with my cravings, especially my addiction to alcohol. When I began the diet, I weighed 142 pounds (5'3" and age 45). In six weeks I lost fourteen pounds. I have a lot more energy, am sleeping better, feel much more relaxed, have improved digestion/elimination, and my overall well-being has improved. Before I began the program, I felt as if I was headed toward having a heart attack (seriously). My lifestyle and eating habits were horrible. Now I've cleaned up my act and feel like a new person. My family cannot believe the change! Thank you so much for helping me become a 'new and improved' person."

Self-reported outcomes from the Blood Type Diet Web site (www.dadamo.com)

AVING BLOOD TYPE A PLACES YOU AT SPECIAL RISK FOR cardiovascular disease. This fact is borne out in numerous studies showing a clear-cut association between being Blood Type A and an increased risk for heart disease. Blood Type A individuals have higher rates of heart attack across all age groups, genders, and ethnic and national groups.

Several Blood Type A–specific characteristics are responsible for this higher risk. A number of studies show that Blood Types A and AB are more likely to be at risk of heart disease and death by virtue of elevated cholesterol. The underlying reason for this tendency is Blood Type A's difficulty breaking down dietary fats due to lower levels of the enzyme responsible for this function, intestinal alkaline phosphatase.

High levels of the blood clotting factor, factor VIII, have been linked to coronary artery disease, and this may in part explain why it shows a higher rate of occurrence in Blood Type A. Greater blood viscosity (thickness) increases the potential for developing arterial blood clots.

Blood Type A individuals have a susceptibility to arterial inflammation—a condition usually considered the first stage of coronary artery disease and arteriosclerosis. They tend to have higher levels of binding sites (selectins) that the white blood cells of the immune system use to attach to the vessel walls as a prelude to moving into the tissues. When this process is out of control, the delicate lining of the blood vessels can become damaged, thus attracting platelets (specialized clotting cells), and eventually resulting in calcification and narrowing of the opening, or lumen. Not only are these binding sites more active in Blood Type A individuals, their activities are enhanced by the high levels of factor VII and cholesterol that are characteristic of Blood Type A.

Blood Type A has another challenge to cardiac health—the effects of high levels of the stress hormone cortisol, and difficulty clearing it from the body once the stressful event has passed. That means Blood Type A tends to be in a physiological state of stress, even when external circumstances are not stressful.

Excessive or prolonged release of cortisol has been linked to heart

---

Blood Type A

TOP TWELVE HEART-HEALTHY FOODS

1. Soy foods
2. Richly oiled cold-water fish
3. Olive oil
4. Walnuts
5. Mushrooms (maitake/silver dollar)
6. Garlic
7. Leafy green vegetables
8. Blueberries, blackberries, cherries
9. Pineapple
10. Ginger
11. Herbal teas (chamomile, dandelion, hawthorn)
12. Green tea

---

disease, hypertension, insulin resistance, and obesity. It is also known to increase the viscosity of blood. The Mayo Clinic has reported that psychological stress is the strongest predictor of recurrent heart attacks and cardiac death among patients being treated for their first heart attacks. Adjustments for other factors associated with recurrent heart attacks or early rehospitalization did not reduce the strength or significance of stress as a leading factor.

Like other blood type–specific factors, high cortisol can be controlled with the Blood Type Diet and lifestyle adjustments.

Blood Type A: The Foods

THE BLOOD TYPE A Cardiovascular Diet is specifically adapted for the prevention and management of cardiovascular disease. A new category, **Super Beneficial**, highlights powerful disease-fighting foods for Blood Type A. The **Neutral** category has also been adjusted to de-emphasize foods that are less advantageous for you. Foods designated **Neutral: Allowed Infrequently** should be minimized or avoided entirely.

Food Values

SUPER BENEFICIAL	Foods that are known to have specific disease-fighting qualities for your blood type.
BENEFICIAL	Foods with components that enhance the metabolic, immune, or structural health of you blood type.
NEUTRAL: Allowed Infrequently	Foods that normally have no direct type effect but may impede your progress when consumed regularly.
AVOID	Foods with components that are harmful to your blood type.

Your secretor status can influence your ability to fully digest and metabolize certain foods, so various adjustments in the values are made for non-secretors. If you do not know your secretor type, the odds are that you can safely use the "secretor" values, since the majority of the population (approximately 80 percent) are secretors. However, I urge you to get tested, since the variations are important for non-secretors who want to maximize the effectiveness of the Blood Type Diet.

The food charts are divided into three sections. The top of the chart suggests the average portion size and quantity per week or day, according to secretor status. These recommendations do *not* apply to the category **Neutral: Allowed Infrequently**; those foods should be eaten rarely, if at all. The charts also indicate differences in frequency for some foods, based on ethnic heritage. It has been my experience that this factor has an impact upon the individual's ability to fully digest certain foods. For the purposes of blood type food choices, persons of Hispanic heritage should follow the recommendations for Caucasians; North American Native peoples should follow the recommendations for Asians.

The middle section of the chart gives the food values. The bottom section lists variants based on secretor status.

For your convenience, we have included a number of product names (Ezekiel 4:9 bread, Worcestershire sauce, etc.). However, keep in mind that commercial formulations vary among brands and regions. Even though a product may be listed as acceptable for you, always check its ingredients; do not use products that contain **Avoid** ingredients for your blood type. Of course, you may choose to make your own version of commercial products, such as bread and mayonnaise, using ingredients that suit your blood type. There are hundreds of delicious recipes for every blood type available on our Web site (www.dadamo. com), and in the book *Cook Right 4 Your Type: The Practical Kitchen Companion to* Eat Right 4 Your Type.

Meat/Poultry

Blood Type A lacks some of the enzymes and stomach acids needed to effectively digest animal protein. For this reason, you should derive most of your protein from non-meat sources. High animal protein consumption can aggravate the Blood Type A tendency toward high LDL cholesterol, as well as accelerated blood clotting, which can cause arterial damage. When you do eat meat or fowl, stick to small portions. Choose only the highest quality (preferably grass-fed) chemical-, antibiotic-, and pesticide-free low-fat meats and poultry.

BLOOD TYPE A: MEAT/POULTRY			
Portion: 4–6 oz (men); 2–5 oz (women and children)			
	African	Caucasian	Asian
Secretor	0–2	0–3	0–3
Non-Secretor	2–5	2–4	2–3
		Times per week	

SUPER BENEFICIAL	BENEFICIAL	NEUTRAL: Allowed Frequently	NEUTRAL: Allowed Infrequently	AVOID
		Chicken		All commercially processed meats
		Cornish hen		Bacon/Ham/Pork
		Grouse		Beef
		Guinea hen		Buffalo
		Ostrich		Duck
		Squab		Goat
		Turkey		Goose
				Heart (beef)
				Horse
				Lamb
				Liver (calf)
				Mutton
				Partridge
				Pheasant
				Quail
				Rabbit
				Squirrel
				Sweetbreads
				Turtle
				Veal
				Venison

Special Variants: *Non-Secretor* BENEFICIAL: turkey; NEUTRAL (Allowed Frequently): duck, goat, goose, lamb, mutton, partridge, pheasant, quail, rabbit, turtle.

Fish/Seafood

Fish and seafood represent a nutrient-rich source of protein for Blood Type A. Because of this, fish is probably the best food for maintaining cardiovascular health. Many kinds of fish are rich in omega series fatty acids, which can help to increase HDL ("good") cholesterol and lower homocysteine levels. Fish are also a good source of selenium, a nutrient essential to controlling inflammation, by way of its effects on selections.

BLOOD TYPE A: FISH/SEAFOOD			
Portion: 4–6 oz (men); 2–5 oz (women and children)			
	African	Caucasian	Asian
Secretor	1–3	1–3	1–3
Non-Secretor	2–5	2–5	2–4
			Times per week

SUPER BENEFICIAL	BENEFICIAL	NEUTRAL: Allowed Frequently	NEUTRAL: Allowed Infrequently	AVOID
Cod	Carp	Abalone		Anchovy
Red snapper	Mackerel	Bass (sea)		Barracuda
Salmon	Monkfish	Bullhead		Bass (bluegill/striped)
Sardine	Perch (silver/yellow)	Butterfish		Beluga
Trout (rainbow)	Pickerel	Croaker		Bluefish
	Pollock	Cusk		Catfish
	Snail (*Helix pomatia*/escargot)	Drum		Caviar (sturgeon)
	Trout (sea)	Halfmoon fish		Clam
	Whitefish	Mahi-mahi		Conch
	Whiting	Mullet		Crab
		Muskellunge		Crayfish
		Orange roughy		Eel
		Parrot fish		Flounder

SUPER BENEFICIAL	BENEFICIAL	NEUTRAL: Allowed Frequently	NEUTRAL: Allowed Infrequently	AVOID
		Perch (white)		Frog
		Pike		Gray sole
		Pompano		Grouper
		Porgy		Haddock
		Rosefish		Hake
		Sailfish		Halibut
		Salmon roe		Harvest fish
		Scrod		Herring (fresh/ pickled/ smoked)
		Shark		
		Smelt		
		Sturgeon		Lobster
		Sucker		Mussels
		Sunfish		Octopus
		Swordfish		Opaleye
		Tilapia		Oyster
		Trout (brook)		Salmon (smoked)
		Tuna		Scallop
		Weakfish		Scup
		Yellowtail		Shad
				Shrimp
				Sole
				Squid (calamari)
				Tilefish

Special Variants: *Non-Secretor* BENEFICIAL: chub, cusk, drum, halfmoon fish, harvest fish, mullet, muskellunge, perch (white), pompano, rosefish, sailfish, sucker, swordfish, trout (brook); NEUTRAL (Allowed Frequently): anchovy, bass (bluegill), beluga, bluefish, caviar (sturgeon), flounder, frog, gray sole, grouper, haddock, hake, halibut, herring (fresh), mussels, octopus, opaleye, scallop, scup, shad, tilefish.

Dairy/Eggs

Dairy products can be used in small quantities by Blood Type A, especially if you limit them to cultured foods, such as yogurt and kefir. Eggs can be consumed a couple of times a week—slightly more often for non-secretors. They are a good source of docosahexaenoic acid (DHA). However, fish is a better source of DHA than eggs, since Blood Type A is associated with greater sensitivity to dietary sources of cholesterol than the other blood types.

Do your best to find eggs and dairy products that meet organic standards.

BLOOD TYPE A: EGGS			
Portion: 1 egg			
	African	Caucasian	Asian
Secretor	1–3	1–3	1–3
Non-Secretor	2–3	2–5	2–4
		Times per week	

BLOOD TYPE A: MILK AND YOGURT			
Portion: 4–6 oz (men); 2–5 oz (women and children)			
	African	Caucasian	Asian
Secretor	0–1	1–3	0–3
Non-Secretor	0–1	1–2	0–2
		Times per week	

BLOOD TYPE A: CHEESE			
Portion: 3 oz (men); 2 oz (women and children)			
	African	Caucasian	Asian
Secretor	0–2	1–3	0–2
Non-Secretor	0	0–1	0–1
		Times per week	

SUPER BENEFICIAL	BENEFICIAL	NEUTRAL: Allowed Frequently	NEUTRAL: Allowed Infrequently	AVOID
		Egg (chicken/ duck/ goose/ quail)	Feta	American cheese
		Farmer cheese	Goat cheese	Blue cheese
		Ghee (clarified butter)	Milk (goat)	Brie
		Kefir	Sour cream	Butter
		Mozzarella		Buttermilk
		Paneer		Camembert
		Ricotta		Casein
		Yogurt		Cheddar
				Colby
				Cottage cheese
				Cream cheese
				Edam
				Emmenthal
				Gouda
				Gruyère
				Half-and-half
				Ice cream
				Jarlsberg
				Milk (cow)
				Monterey Jack
				Muenster
				Neufchâtel
				Parmesan
				Provolone
				Sherbet
				Swiss cheese
				Whey

Special Variants: *Non-Secretor* NEUTRAL (Allowed Frequently): cottage cheese, whey; AVOID: milk (goat), sour cream.

Oils

In general, Blood Type A does best on monounsaturated oils (such as olive oil) and oils rich in omega series fatty acids (such as flax oil). Olive oil's cardiovascular benefits are related to its component squalene, which enhances cholesterol synthesis.

BLOOD TYPE A: OILS			
Portion: 1 tblsp			
	African	Caucasian	Asian
Secretor	5–8	5–8	5–8
Non-Secretor	3–7	3–7	3–6
		Times per week	

SUPER BENEFICIAL	BENEFICIAL	NEUTRAL: Allowed Frequently	NEUTRAL: Allowed Infrequently	AVOID
Flax (linseed) Olive	Black currant seed Walnut	Almond Avocado Borage seed Cod liver Evening primrose Safflower Sesame Soy Sunflower Wheat germ	Canola	Castor Coconut Corn Cottonseed Peanut

Special Variants: *Non-Secretor* BENEFICIAL cod liver, sesame; NEUTRAL (Allowed Frequently): peanut; AVOID: safflower.

Nuts and Seeds

Nuts and seeds can serve as an important secondary source of protein for Blood Type A. Walnuts and peanuts can aid in blood sugar regulation, and walnuts can help lower LDL cholesterol. Flax (linseed) is an excellent source of fiber and is also known to protect the arteries, inhibit blood clots, lower blood pressure and overall cholesterol, and reduce the risk of heart attack and stroke.

BLOOD TYPE A: NUTS AND SEEDS			
Portion: Whole (handful); Nut Butters (2 tblsp)			
	African	Caucasian	Asian
Secretor	4–7	4–7	4–7
Non-Secretor	5–7	5–7	5–7
			Times per week

SUPER BENEFICIAL	BENEFICIAL	NEUTRAL: Allowed Frequently	NEUTRAL: Allowed Infrequently	AVOID
Flax (linseed)	Pumpkin seed	Almond	Safflower seed	Brazil nut
Peanut		Almond butter	Sesame butter (tahini)	Cashew
Peanut butter		Almond cheese	Sesame seed	Pistachio
Walnut (black/English)		Almond milk		
		Beechnut		
		Butternut		
		Chestnut		
		Filbert (hazelnut)		
		Hickory nut		
		Litchi		
		Macadamia nut		
		Pecan		

SUPER BENEFICIAL	BENEFICIAL	NEUTRAL: Allowed Frequently	NEUTRAL: Allowed Infrequently	AVOID
		Pignolia (pine nut)		
		Poppy seed		
		Sunflower butter		
		Sunflower seed		

Special Variants: *Non-Secretor* AVOID: safflower seed, sunflower seed.

Beans and Legumes

Blood Type A does well on vegetable proteins found in many beans and legumes, although some beans contain problematic lectins. In general, this category, along with appropriate choices of seafood, is more than sufficient to build active tissue mass for Blood Type A. The BENEFICIAL and SUPER BENEFICIAL beans are all excellent sources of essential amino acids and can support cardiovascular health and blood sugar regulation. In particular, Blood Type A thrives on soy foods, which not only have cardiovascular benefits (soy isoflavones are effective blockers of selectin activity, a marker of blood vessel inflammation), but are essential to healthy immune system function for Blood Type A. A number of studies have shown that the regular consumption of soy protein significantly reduces LDL cholesterol, especially for individuals with extremely high levels (over 355 mg/dL).

BLOOD TYPE A: BEANS AND LEGUMES			
Portion: 1 cup (cooked)			
	African	Caucasian	Asian
Secretor	5–7	5–7	5–7
Non-Secretor	3–5	3–5	3–5
	Times per week		

SUPER BENEFICIAL	BENEFICIAL	NEUTRAL: Allowed Frequently	NEUTRAL: Allowed Infrequently	AVOID
Miso	Adzuki bean	Cannellini bean		Copper bean
Soy bean	Bean (green/snap/string)	Jicama bean		Garbanzo (chickpea)
Soy cheese		Mung bean/sprouts		Kidney bean
Soy milk				Lima bean
Tempeh	Black bean	Northern bean		Navy bean
Tofu	Black-eyed pea	Pea (green/pod/snow)		Tamarind bean
	Fava (broad) bean	White bean		
	Lentil (all)			
	Pinto bean			

Special Variants: *Non-Secretor* NEUTRAL (Allowed Frequently): adzuki bean, bean (green/snap/string), black bean, black-eyed pea, copper bean, fava (broad) bean, kidney bean, navy bean, soy bean and products.

Grains and Starches

If you have heart disease, diabetes, metabolic syndrome, or are overweight, limit your intake of wheat and corn; their lectins can exert an insulinlike effect, lowering active tissue mass and increasing total body fat. Note, however, that the lectin in wheat can often be milled out of the grain or destroyed by sprouting. Examples are sprouted seed breads, such as Essene and Ezekiel, usually found in the freezer section of your health-food store. The gluten lectins, principally found in the seed coats, are destroyed in the sprouting process. Unlike many commercially sprouted breads, Essene and Ezekiel are "live" foods, with many beneficial enzymes intact.

BLOOD TYPE A: GRAINS AND STARCHES			
Portion: ½ cup dry (grains or pastas); 1 muffin; 2 slices of bread			
	African	Caucasian	Asian
Secretor	7–10	7–9	7–10
Non-Secretor	5–7	5–7	5–7
		Times per week	

SUPER BENEFICIAL	BENEFICIAL	NEUTRAL: Allowed Frequently	NEUTRAL: Allowed Infrequently	AVOID
	Amaranth	Barley	Cornmeal	Teff
	Buckwheat	Kamut	Couscous	Wheat bran
	Essene bread (manna)	Quinoa	Grits	Wheat germ
	Ezekiel 4:9 bread	Rice (wild)	Millet	
	Oat bran	Rice cake	Popcorn	
	Oat flour	Rice flour/ products	Tapioca	
	Oatmeal	Rice milk	Wheat (whole)	
	Rice (whole)	Rye flour/ products		
	Rice bran	Sorghum		
	Rye (whole)	Spelt (whole)		
	Soba noodles (100% buck-wheat)	Spelt flour/ products		
	Soy flour/ products	Wheat (refined/ un-bleached)		
		Wheat (semolina)		
		Wheat (white flour)		

SUPER BENEFICIAL	BENEFICIAL	NEUTRAL: Allowed Frequently	NEUTRAL: Allowed Infrequently	AVOID
		100% sprouted grain products (except Essene, Ezekiel)		

Special Variants: *Non-Secretor* NEUTRAL (Allowed Frequently): buckwheat, Ezekiel bread, oat (all), soba noodles (100% buckwheat), soy flour/products, teff; AVOID: cornmeal, couscous, grits, popcorn, wheat (all).

Vegetables

Vegetables provide a rich source of antioxidants and fiber and are crucial to intestinal health. Garlic is SUPER BENEFICIAL for Blood Type A because of its ability to reduce excess blood clotting factors. Onions are also SUPER BENEFICIAL. They contain significant amounts of the antioxidant quercetin, as well as beneficial polysaccharides known to aid blood sugar regulation. Green, leafy vegetables, such as collards, escarole, rappini, spinach, and Swiss chard, are good sources of magnesium, a mineral often found lacking in people with high cholesterol and triglyceride levels. Artichoke and dandelion aid liver and gallbladder functions, which are sometimes impaired in Blood Type A. Many vegetables are rich in potassium, which helps reduce "water weight." The common white domestic ("silver dollar") mushroom contains lectins that aid metabolic function.

Tomatoes contain a lectin that reacts with the saliva and digestive juices of Blood Type A secretors, although it does not appear to react with non-secretors. Yams are typically high in the amino acid phenylalanine, which inactivates intestinal alkaline phosphatase (already quite low in Blood Type A) and should be avoided.

An item's value also applies to its juice, unless otherwise noted.

BLOOD TYPE A: VEGETABLES			
Portion: 1 cup, prepared (cooked or raw)			
	African	Caucasian	Asian
Secretor Super/ Beneficials	Unlimited	Unlimited	Unlimited
Secretor Neutrals	2–5	2–5	2–5
Non-Secretor Super/ Beneficials	Unlimited	Unlimited	Unlimited
Non-Secretor Neutrals	2–3	2–3	2–3
	Times per day		

SUPER BENEFICIAL	BENEFICIAL	NEUTRAL: Allowed Frequently	NEUTRAL: Allowed Infrequently	AVOID
Artichoke	Alfalfa	Arugula	Corn	Cabbage
Broccoli	sprouts	Asparagus	Olive	Eggplant
Collards	Aloe	Asparagus	(green)	Mushroom
Dandelion	Beet	pea	Pickles (in	(shiitake)
Escarole	Beet greens	Bamboo	brine)	Olive
Garlic	Carrot	shoot	Squash (all)	(black/
Mushroom	Celery	Beet		Greek/
(maitake/	Chicory	Bok choy		Spanish)
silver	Horseradish	Brussels		Peppers (all)
dollar)	Kale	sprouts		Pickles (in
Onion (all)	Kohlrabi	Cabbage		vinegar)
Rappini	Leek	(juice)*		Potato
(broccoli	Lettuce	Cauli-		Potato
rabe)	(Romaine)	flower		(sweet)
Spinach	Okra	Celeriac		Rhubarb
Swiss	Parsnip	Cucumber		Tomato
chard	Pumpkin	Daikon		Yam
	Turnip	radish		Yucca
		Endive		
		Fennel		

SUPER BENEFICIAL	BENEFICIAL	NEUTRAL: Allowed Frequently	NEUTRAL: Allowed Infrequently	AVOID
		Fiddlehead fern		
		Lettuce (except Romaine)		
		Mushroom (abalone/ enoki/ oyster/ porto- bello/ straw/ tree ear)		
		Mustard greens		
		Oyster plant		
		Poi		
		Radicchio		
		Radish/ sprouts		
		Rutabaga		
		Scallion		
		Seaweeds		
		Shallot		
		Taro		
		Water chestnut		
		Watercress		
		Zucchini		

Special Variants: *Non-Secretor* NEUTRAL (Allowed Frequently): alfalfa sprouts, aloe, carrot, celery, eggplant, fennel, garlic, horseradish, lettuce (Romaine), mushroom (maitake/shiitake), peppers (all), potato (sweet), rappini, taro, tomato; AVOID: agar, cabbage (juice), mushroom (silver dollar), olive (green), pickles (in brine).

*To obtain the benefits of cabbage juice, it must be consumed within one minute of juicing.

Fruits and Fruit Juices

Fruits are rich in antioxidants, and many, such as blueberries, cherries, and blackberries, contain polysaccharides that aid weight loss by tempering the effects of insulin. Many fruits, such as pineapple, help normalize the balance of water, thus preventing edema. Lemon is an effective clot inhibitor for Blood Type A. Other fruits, such as red grapefruit and guava, replace tomatoes as rich sources of the antioxidant lycopene.

Grapefruit juice is a well-documented culprit in many food-drug interactions. Grapefruit juice can inhibit the metabolism of certain heart and blood pressure drugs, including Nifedipine, Verapamil, and Lovastatin. Many readers have reported cautionary warnings of grapefruit's interaction appearing on Coumadin (warfarin prescriptions; blood thinners). There is no evidence in the medical literature to support this interaction. Grapefruit's effect on warfarin is insignificant.

An item's value also applies to its juice, unless otherwise noted.

BLOOD TYPE A: FRUITS AND FRUIT JUICES			
Portion: 1 cup			
	African	Caucasian	Asian
Secretor	2–4	3–4	3–4
Non-Secretor	2–3	2–3	2–3
			Times per day

SUPER BENEFICIAL	BENEFICIAL	NEUTRAL: Allowed Frequently	NEUTRAL: Allowed Infrequently	AVOID
Blackberry	Apricot	Apple	Currant	Banana
Blueberry	Boysen-	Asian pear	Date	Bitter melon
Cherry	berry	Avocado	Grape (all)	Coconut
Lemon	Cranberry	Breadfruit	Pome-	Honeydew
Pineapple	Fig (fresh/	Canang	granate	Mango
Plum	dried)	melon	Quince	Orange
Prune	Grapefruit	Cantaloupe	Raisin	Papaya

SUPER BENEFICIAL	BENEFICIAL	NEUTRAL: Allowed Frequently	NEUTRAL: Allowed Infrequently	AVOID
	Lime	Casaba melon	Star fruit (carambola)	Plantain
		Christmas melon	Strawberry	Tangerine
		Cranberry (juice)		
		Crenshaw melon		
		Dewberry		
		Elderberry (dark blue/purple		
		Gooseberry		
		Guava		
		Kiwi		
		Kumquat		
		Loganberry		
		Mulberry		
		Muskmelon		
		Nectarine		
		Peach		
		Pear		
		Persian melon		
		Persimmon		
		Prickly pear		
		Raspberry		
		Sago palm		
		Spanish melon		
		Watermelon		
		Youngberry		

Special Variants: *Non-Secretor* BENEFICIAL: cranberry (juice), elderberry (dark blue/purple) watermelon; NEUTRAL (Allowed Frequently): banana, coconut, lime, mango, plantain, tangerine; AVOID: cantaloupe, casaba melon.

Spices/Condiments/Sweeteners

Many spices have mild to moderate medicinal properties, often by influencing the levels of bacteria in the lower colon. Turmeric contains a powerful phytochemical called curcumin, which helps improve liver function. Coriander seeds have been shown to enhance the synthesis of bile acid by the liver, lowering overall cholesterol. They have also been shown to increase HDL ("good") cholesterol. Fenugreek can help in the treatment of atherosclerosis.

Many common food additives, such as guar gum and carrageenan, should be avoided as they can enhance the effects of lectins found in other foods.

SUPER BENEFICIAL	BENEFICIAL	NEUTRAL: Allowed Frequently	NEUTRAL: Allowed Infrequently	AVOID
Coriander seeds	Barley malt	Agar	Brown rice syrup	Aspartame
Fenugreek	Horse-radish	Allspice	Chocolate	Capers
Garlic	Molasses (black-strap)	Almond extract	Cornstarch	Carra-geenan
Ginger	Mustard (dry)	Anise	Corn syrup	Chili powder
Turmeric	Parsley	Apple pectin	Dextrose	Gelatin (except veg-sourced)
	Soy sauce	Arrowroot	Fructose	Gums (acacia/Arabic/guar)
	Tamari (wheat-free)	Basil	Guarana	Juniper
		Bay leaf	Honey	Ketchup
		Bergamot	Maltodex-trin	Mayonnaise
		Caraway	Maple syrup	MSG
		Cardamon	Rice syrup	Pepper (black/white)
		Carob	Senna	
		Chervil	Sugar (brown/white)	
		Chive		
		Cilantro (corian-der leaf)		

SUPER BENEFICIAL	BENEFICIAL	NEUTRAL: Allowed Frequently	NEUTRAL: Allowed Infrequently	AVOID
		Cinnamon		Pepper (cayenne)
		Clove		Pepper (peppercorn/ red flakes)
		Cream of tartar		
		Cumin		Pickles/ relish
		Dill		Sucanat
		Invert sugar		Vinegar (all)
		Licorice root*		Wintergreen
		Mace		Worcester- shire sauce
		Marjoram		
		Mint (all)		
		Molasses		
		Nutmeg		
		Oregano		
		Paprika		
		Rosemary		
		Saffron		
		Sage		
		Savory		
		Sea salt		
		Seaweeds		
		Stevia		
		Tamarind		
		Tarragon		
		Thyme		
		Vanilla		
		Vegetable glycerine		

SUPER BENEFICIAL	BENEFICIAL	NEUTRAL: Allowed Frequently	NEUTRAL: Allowed Infrequently	AVOID
		Yeast (baker's/ brewer's)		

Special Variants: *Non-Secretor* BENEFICIAL: cilantro (coriander leaf), yeast (brewer's); NEUTRAL (Allowed Frequently): barley malt, chili powder, parsley, turmeric, soy sauce, tamari (wheat-free), wintergreen; AVOID: agar, cornstarch, corn syrup, senna, dextrose, maltodextrin, rice syrup, sugar (brown/white).

*Do not use if you have high blood pressure.

Herbal Teas

Herbal teas can provide medicinal benefits, and several are SUPER BENEFICIAL for Blood Type A cardiovascular health. Hawthorn improves coronary function, lowers blood pressure, and eases angina. Ginseng helps reduce stress and improve overall cardiac health. Ginger and ginkgo biloba help reduce the viscosity of blood. Chamomile and holy basil help reduce stress by modulating coritsol. Dandelion improves liver function.

SUPER BENEFICIAL	BENEFICIAL	NEUTRAL: Allowed Frequently	NEUTRAL: Allowed Infrequently	AVOID
Chamomile	Alfalfa	Chickweed	Hops	Catnip
Dandelion	Aloe	Coltsfoot	Senna	Cayenne
Fenugreek	Burdock	Dong quai		Corn silk
Ginger	Echinacea	Elderberry		Red clover
Ginkgo biloba	Gentian	Goldenseal		Rhubarb
Ginseng	Milk thistle	Horehound		Yellow dock
Hawthorn	Parsley	Licorice root*		
Holy basil	Rosehip	Linden		
	Slippery elm	Mulberry		

SUPER BENEFICIAL	BENEFICIAL	NEUTRAL: Allowed Frequently	NEUTRAL: Allowed Infrequently	AVOID
	St. John's wort	Mullein		
	Stone root	Peppermint		
	Valerian	Raspberry leaf		
		Sage		
		Sarsaparilla		
		Shepherd's purse		
		Skullcap		
		Spearmint		
		Strawberry leaf		
		Thyme		
		White birch		
		White oak bark		
		Yarrow		

Special Variants: *Non-Secretor* AVOID: senna.

*Avoid if you have high blood pressure.

Miscellaneous Beverages

You may wish to have a glass of wine occasionally; you derive substantial cardiovascular benefits from moderate use. Green tea should be part of every Blood Type A's health plan; the catechins and polyphenols in green tea have been shown to lower LDL (bad cholesterol) by as much as 16 percent. Type As who are not caffeine sensitive might consider having a cup or two of coffee daily; it contains many enzymes also found in soy that can help your endocrine system function more effectively.

SUPER BENEFICIAL	BENEFICIAL	NEUTRAL: Allowed Frequently	NEUTRAL: Allowed Infrequently	AVOID
Tea (green) Wine (red)	Coffee (regular) Coffee (decaf)	Wine (white)		Beer Liquor Seltzer Soda (club) Soda (cola/ diet/misc.) Tea, black (reg/decaf)

Special Variants: *Non-Secretor* BENEFICIAL: wine (white); NEUTRAL (Allowed Frequently): beer, seltzer, soda (club), tea (black: reg/decaf).

Supplements

THE BLOOD TYPE A Diet offers abundant quantities of important nutrients, such as protein and iron. It is important to get as many nutrients as possible from fresh foods and use supplements only to fill in the minor deficiencies in your diet. The following supplement protocols are designed for Blood Type A individuals who are suffering from cardiovascular disease or related conditions.

Note: If you are being treated for a cardiovascular or related condition, consult your doctor before taking any supplements.

Blood Type A: Cardiovascular Protection and Enhancement Protocol

Use this protocol for 4–8 weeks, then discontinue for 2 weeks and restart.

SUPPLEMENT	ACTION	DOSAGE
Coenzyme Q-10 (ubiquinone)	Improves coronary function	30–60 mg daily with meals

SUPPLEMENT	ACTION	DOSAGE
Soy protein powder	Enhances protection of blood vessel lining	Use as directed in a protein drink once daily
Lemon juice	Mild blood-thinning ability.	Juice of ½ lemon daily
Hawthorn (*Crataegus spp.*)	Cardiovascular tonic; improves coronary function; reduces angina	150–250 mg, twice daily

Blood Type A Specific Cardiovascular Treatment Protocols

Use these protocols for 4–8 weeks, then discontinue for 1 week and restart. Protocols can be combined.

Cholesterol Control*

SUPPLEMENT	ACTION	DOSAGE
Garlic	Mild cholesterol-lowering effects	2–4 fresh cloves daily
Soy lecithin	Helps emulsify fats	1–2 tblsp daily
Pantethine (active vitamin B₅)	Lowers cholesterol	500 mg, twice daily

Stress Reduction Protocol

SUPPLEMENT	ACTION	DOSAGE
Chamomile (*Matricaria chamomilla*)	A calming nerve tonic	Herbal tincture; 25 drops in warm water, two to three times daily
Spreading hogweed (*Boerhaavia diffusa*)	Acts as a stress modifier and a liver protector	50–150 mg, twice daily
Holy basil (*Ocimum sanctum*) leaf extract	Lowers cortisol	50 mg, twice daily

Angina Relief Adjunct*

SUPPLEMENT	ACTION	DOSAGE
Coenzyme Q-10 (ubiquinone)	Improves coronary function; reduces angina	30–60 mg daily with meals
Taurine	Increases cardiac output, diminishes angina	500 mg, twice daily
Zinc	Enhances effects of taurine	25 mg, twice daily

Hypertension Control*

SUPPLEMENT	ACTION	DOSAGE
Dandelion (*Taraxacum officinale*)	Mild diuretic; rich in electrolytes	150 mg, twice daily
Hawthorn (*Crataegus spp.*)	Cardiovascular tonic; improves coronary function; reduces angina	150–250 mg, two capsules twice daily
Magnesium	Mild to moderate effects on blood pressure	500 mg, twice daily

Blood Viscosity Control*

SUPPLEMENT	ACTION	DOSAGE
Fish oils	May slow development of heart disease resulting from increased LDL. Omega-3 fatty acids in fish oils discourage platelets from clumping.	1000 mg, once or twice daily
Ginkgo (*Ginkgo biloba*)	Increases cerebral circulation, inhibits platelet aggregation. Not to be taken concurrently with aspirin therapy	Standardized extract: 60 mg daily

*Check with your doctor before beginning this or any other nutritional protocol, especially if you are currently taking prescription medication.

The Exercise Component

FOR BLOOD TYPE A, stress regulation and overall fitness depend on engaging in regular exercises, with an emphasis on calming exercises such as Hatha yoga and T'ai Chi, as well as light aerobic exercise such as walking. These guidelines are perfectly suited to the needs of Blood Type A individuals suffering from cardiovascular disease.

Done properly, yoga can be especially effective for stress reduction. This ancient system of exercise uses special postures to stretch, strengthen, and align the body. Yoga also uses breathing exercises and meditation to focus the mind and promote relaxation. If you have a heart condition, start slowly and be sure to find an instructor who is trained to work with cardiac patients. There are several different styles of yoga, so you need to choose the one that works for your condition. Your primary emphasis should be on breathing, flexibility, and stress reduction.

T'ai Chi, a martial art that is basically a form of moving meditation, can gently improve cardiovascular health. It helps reduce stress, lower blood pressure, and improve mood.

Walking or brisk walking is the ideal aerobic exercise for Blood Type A, especially when you walk outdoors in a quiet, natural setting. Studies consistently show that light aerobic exercise improves cardiovascular function and reduces stress. Physical exercise also promotes lean muscle mass and reduces weight.

The following comprises the ideal exercise regimen for Blood Type A:

EXERCISE	DURATION	FREQUENCY
Hatha yoga	40–50 minutes	3–4 x week
T'ai Chi	40–50 minutes	3–4 x week
Aerobics (low impact)	40–50 minutes	2–3 x week
Treadmill	30 minutes	2–3 x week
Pilates	40–50 minutes	3–4 x week
Weight training (5–10 lb free weights)	15 minutes	2–3 x week

EXERCISE	DURATION	FREQUENCY
Cycling (recumbent bike)	30 minutes	2–3 x week
Swimming	30 minutes	2–3 x week
Brisk walking	45 minutes	2–3 x week

Getting Started: The First Month

IF YOU ARE NEW to the Blood Type Diet, the following guidelines will introduce you to the Blood Type A regimen over a period of one month. Follow these recommendations as closely as possible, using a

Blood Type A Cardiovascular Diet Checklist

Avoid red meat. Low levels of hydrochloric acid and intestinal ☐ alkaline phosphatase make it hard for Blood Type A to digest.

Derive your primary protein from soy foods and other plant ☐ sources.

Include regular portions of richly oiled cold-water fish ☐ every week.

Include modest amounts of cultured dairy foods in your diet, ☐ but limit fresh milk products, which cause excess mucus production.

Eat your beans; beans provide an essential high-protein vegetable source for Blood Type A. ☐

Don't overdo the grains, especially wheat-derived foods. Avoid ☐ wheat if you have a heart condition, diabetes, or are overweight.

Eat lots of BENEFICIAL fruits and vegetables, especially those ☐ high in antioxidants and fiber.

Drink 2 to 3 cups of green tea every day for extra cardiovascular and immune system benefits. ☐

journal to record your personal experiences with the diet. In addition to factors that are measurable in medical tests (EKG, cholesterol levels, blood pressure, and cardiac stress tests), take the time to note changes in your energy levels, sleep patterns, digestion, and overall well-being.

Week 1

Blood Type Diet and Supplements

- Eliminate your most harmful AVOID foods—red meat, most dairy, and negative lectin-containing nuts, beans, and seeds.

- Include your most important BENEFICIAL foods frequently throughout the week. For example, have soy-based foods 5 times, and omega-3-rich fish 3 to 4 times, with lots of BENEFICIAL vegetables and fruit.

- Incorporate at least 1 SUPER BENEFICIAL food into your daily diet. For example, have a bowl of cherries as a snack, or a spinach salad with walnuts.

- Drink 2 to 3 cups of green tea every day.

Exercise Regimen

- Plan to exercise at least 4 days this week, for 45 minutes each day.

  2 days: walking or light aerobic activity

  2 days: yoga or T'ai Chi

- If you experience angina during exercise, consult with a physician. Angina is a warning sign that some of your heart muscle is not getting enough oxygen.

- Use your journal to detail the time, activity, distance, and amount of weight. Note the number of repetitions for each exercise.

■ WEEK 1 SUCCESS STRATEGY ■
Type A Blood Tonic

Although it is not documented in the literature, one of my teachers, the noted naturopath John Bastyr, used to say that the juice of 3 to 4 lemons has a clot-inhibiting action comparable to the drug Coumadin. This is a good tonic for Blood Type As to take first thing in the morning, as it has the added benefit of reducing mucus production, a frequent problem for Type A.

Week 2

Blood Type Diet and Supplements

- Begin to eliminate the next level of AVOID foods—grains, vegetables, and fruits—that react poorly with Type A blood.

- Eat 2 to 3 BENEFICIAL proteins every day, with special emphasis on soy. Eat omega-3-rich fish at least 3 times a week.

- Continue to incorporate SUPER BENEFICIAL foods into your daily diet.

- Choose the NEUTRAL foods listed as Allowed Frequently, over those listed as Allowed Infrequently.

- Manage your mealtimes to aid proper digestion. Avoid eating on the run. Make your meals relaxing, sit-down affairs. Eat slowly and chew thoroughly to encourage digestive secretions.

- Drink a soothing, stress-busting herbal tea, such as chamomile or holy basil, before bedtime.

Exercise Regimen

- Continue to exercise at least 4 days this week, for 45 minutes each day.

  2 days: walking or light aerobic activity

  2 days: yoga or T'ai Chi

- If your work is sedentary, get in the habit of taking a couple of "movement" breaks during the day. Walk around the block or up and down stairs.

■ WEEK 2 SUCCESS STRATEGY ■
Here's to Good Health!

A glass of red wine may be exactly what the doctor ordered, especially if you are not sensitive to alcohol. Researchers analyzed the high-density lipoprotein composition of teetotalers, regular drinkers, and heavy drinkers (most of whom generally drank red wine). They found that HDL cholesterol increased as alcohol consumption increased, and that HDL particles from wine consumption were richer in certain components that can play a protective role in cardiovascular disease. Some of these components may be found in other foods, such as grapes or red grape juice, so if you are sensitive to alcoholic beverages, you may want to investigate these alternatives.

Week 3

Blood Type Diet and Supplements

- When you plan your meals for week 3, choose BENEFICIAL foods to replace NEUTRAL foods whenever possible. For example, choose tofu over chicken, or blueberries over an apple.
- Eliminate all remaining AVOID foods.
- Liberally incorporate SUPER BENEFICIAL foods into your daily diet.
- Drink 2 or 3 cups of green tea every day.

Exercise Regimen

- Continue to exercise at least 4 days this week, for 45 minutes each day.

  2 days: walking or light aerobic activity

  2 days: yoga or T'ai Chi

■ WEEK 3 SUCCESS STRATEGY ■
Chi Breathing

Chi breathing is based on the Taoist concept of Chi Gong, which represents energy as flowing according to certain routes in your body. Positive release is accessible through refining the breath. The calming, stress-relieving effects of this exercise are remarkable. It can be performed by anyone, regardless of age, fitness, or medical condition.

1. Stand comfortably, feet shoulder-width apart, knees slightly bent, arms at your side. Relax your neck and shoulder muscles and focus on your solar plexus (center of the body). It is okay to sway a bit—that's normal.
2. Start to rock back and forth gently. Inhale deeply as you rock forward onto the balls of your feet; exhale as you rock backward onto your heels.
3. As you inhale, lift your relaxed arms up and forward, keeping them relaxed and slightly bent. As you exhale, let your arms float down. Imagine that your hands are pulsing around an imaginary ball of energy.
4. Repeat, gradually refining the rhythm and developing the ability to "drop" your breath from the lungs to the solar plexus.

5. Repeat four to five times, then relax, letting your hands drop to your sides and closing your eyes. Concentrate on feeling relaxed and centered.

Week 4

Blood Type Diet and Supplements

- Continue at the week 3 level, focusing on BENEFICIAL and SUPER BENEFICIAL foods.
- Evaluate the first 4 weeks and make adjustments.

Exercise Regimen

- Continue at the week 3 level.
- Review your progress, noting in your journal improvements in strength and flexibility. Determine which exercise regimen has worked for you, including time of day, setting, and activity level.

■ WEEK 4 SUCCESS STRATEGY ■
Timing Is Everything

For Blood Type A, the timing of your meals can be almost as important as what you eat. This is particularly true if you're trying to lose weight. The following are helpful guidelines:

- Never skip meals. You won't be "saving" calories, as the metabolic reaction will foil your efforts.
- Make breakfast your most important protein-rich meal of the day. The result will be an efficient metabolism all day long.
- Eat on a sliding scale: big breakfast, medium lunch, small dinner.
- Resist the late-night munchies, but if you have problems regulating blood sugar, have a small protein snack—yogurt or soy milk—before bedtime.

A Final Word

IN SUMMARY, the secret to fighting cardiovascular disease with the Blood Type A Diet involves:

1. Decreasing arterial and venous inflammation by eating a diet rich in soy protein, healthy seafood, and green vegetables.
2. Minimizing consumption of the insulin-mimicking lectins abundant in AVOID beans, grains, and vegetables, which can contribute to metabolic syndrome, a precursor to heart disease.
3. Improving your metabolic health, lowering your cholesterol, controlling your blood pressure, improving liver function, and lowering your risk for heart disease by avoiding red meat and high-fat foods.
4. Reducing cortisol levels by engaging in regular exercise— and by not overdoing it.
5. Using supplements intelligently to block the effect of insulin-mimicking lectins, provide antioxidant support, and keep the blood flowing easily.

Blood Type

B

BLOOD TYPE B DIET OUTCOME: STUDIES IN SUCCESS

"My husband and I are both Blood Type B. When we started the diet, my hypoglycemia disappeared almost overnight, and my husband's sinuses and snoring cleared up. I am a registered/licensed dietitian specializing in complementary care, so I see lots of chronic pain and inflammatory conditions that allopathic medicine hasn't helped. Without exception, my clients who use the Blood Type Diet regularly experience dramatic improvement in less than thirty days. Their physicians ask them how they were able to decrease their pain meds, or how they dropped their cholesterol 150 points. They are amazed at the results. So am I. I will continue to follow and recommend the Blood Type Diet to everyone. My dad, at 65, says he feels so good he's guilty (but he gets over it)."

BLOOD TYPE B DIET OUTCOME: ALIVE AGAIN

"Since going on the Blood Type B Diet, I have no more insomnia, my cholesterol has dropped 50 points, and my HDL/LDL ratios are great. I feel alive again. I followed a vegetarian diet for 15 years after open heart surgery, and took every cholesterol medicine available. I couldn't sleep without medication. Meditation was nearly impossible with no sleep, and staying centered was a real problem. I found myself reacting rather than listening. It is so good to be still again."

Self-reported outcomes from the Blood Type Diet Web site (www.dadamo.com)

N GENERAL, A BLOOD TYPE B INDIVIDUAL LIVING RIGHT FOR his or her type tends to have fewer risk factors for cardiovascular disease than the other blood types—and those that you do have are somewhat controllable.

The primary challenges faced by Blood Type B involve a sensitivity to B-specific lectins in certain foods, which can impair fat metabolism, and the tendency to produce higher than normal levels of the hormone cortisol in situations of stress.

Another potential cardiovascular challenge for Blood Type B individuals involves the ineffective regulation of nitric oxide, a chemical released by the cells lining the artery walls. Nitric oxide allows blood vessels to relax and open up.

Finally, Blood Type B arteries can be damaged by high levels of homocysteine, an amino acid (building block of protein) that is produced in the human body. Homocysteine may irritate blood vessels,

---

Blood Type B

TOP THIRTEEN HEART-HEALTHY FOODS

1. Lean, organic lamb and mutton
2. Richly oiled cold-water fish
3. Cultured dairy foods (yogurt, kefir)
4. Olive oil
5. Black walnuts
6. Shiitake mushrooms
7. Broccoli
8. Collards, kale, mustard greens
9. Pineapple
10. Cranberries
11. Herbal teas: dandelion, ginseng, licorice root
12. Turmeric
13. Green tea

leading to blockages in the arteries. High homocysteine levels in the blood can also cause cholesterol to change to a form that is more damaging to arteries (called oxidized LDL). Blood Type B individuals can raise their homocysteine levels when they consume the wrong kinds of animal protein.

You will have to be alert to certain idiosyncratic variations. For example, if you are lactose intolerant, you'll need to favor cultured dairy products (such as kefir and yogurt), introduce dairy foods very gradually, and perhaps utilize lactase enzyme supplements, at least initially.

Like Blood Type O, Blood Type B receives some protection from heart disease because of high levels of intestinal alkaline phosphatase, and lower levels of certain blood clotting factors that discourage dangerous clot formation. As we discussed in chapter 2, intestinal alkaline phosphatase is an enzyme manufactured in the small intestine, which has the primary function of splitting dietary cholesterol and fats, aiding their efficient digestion and metabolism. Blood Type B has naturally high levels of this enzyme, and well-chosen protein consumption increases the levels even further.

Stress on the Heart

Blood Type B has somewhat higher than normal levels of the stress hormone cortisol, placing you in a physiological state of stress, even when external circumstances are not stressful. Excessive or prolonged release of cortisol has been linked to heart disease, hypertension, insulin resistance, and obesity. It is also known to increase the viscosity of blood. The Mayo Clinic has reported that psychological stress is the strongest predictor of recurrent heart attacks and cardiac death among patients being treated for their first heart attacks. Adjustments for other factors associated with recurrent heart attacks or early rehospitalization did not reduce the strength or significance of stress as a leading factor.

Like other blood type–specific factors, high cortisol can be controlled with the Blood Type Diet and lifestyle adjustments.

Blood Type B: The Foods

The Blood Type B Cardiovascular Diet is specifically adapted for the prevention and management of cardiovascular disease. A new category, **Super Beneficial**, highlights powerful disease-fighting foods for Blood Type B. The **Neutral** category has also been adjusted to de-emphasize foods that are less advantageous for you. Foods designated **Neutral: Allowed Infrequently** should be minimized or avoided entirely.

Food Values

SUPER BENEFICIAL	Foods that are known to have specific disease-fighting qualities for your blood type.
BENEFICIAL	Foods with components that enhance the metabolic, immune, or structural health of you blood type.
NEUTRAL: **Aliowed Infrequently**	Foods that normally have no direct type effect but may impede your progress when consumed regularly.
AVOID	Foods with components that are harmful to your blood type.

Your secretor status can influence your ability to fully digest and metabolize certain foods, so various adjustments in the values are made for non-secretors. If you do not know your secretor type, the odds are that you can safely use the "secretor" values, since the majority of the population (approximately 80 percent) are secretors. However, I urge you to get tested, since the variations are important for non-secretors who want to maximize the effectiveness of the Blood Type Diet.

The food charts are divided into three sections. The top of the chart suggests the average portion size and quantity per week or day, according to secretor status. These recommendations do *not* apply to the category **Neutral: Allowed Infrequently**; those foods should be eaten rarely, if at all. The charts also indicate differences in frequency for some foods based on ethnic heritage. It has been my experience that this factor has an impact upon the individual's ability to fully digest certain foods. For the purposes of blood type food choices, persons of Hispanic heritage should follow the recommendations for Caucasians; North American Native peoples should follow the recommendations for Asians.

The middle section of the chart gives the food values. The bottom section lists variants based on secretor status.

For your convenience, we have included a number of product names (Ezekiel 4:9 bread, Worcestershire sauce, etc.). However, keep in mind that commercial formulations vary among brands and regions. Even though a product may be listed as acceptable for you, always check its ingredients; do not use products that contain **Avoid** ingredients for your blood type. Of course, you may choose to make your own version of commercial products, such as bread and mayonnaise, using ingredients that suit your blood type. There are hundreds of delicious recipes for every blood type available on our Web site (www.dadamo. com), and in the book *Cook Right 4 Your Type: The Practical Kitchen Companion to* Eat Right 4 Your Type.

Meat/Poultry

Blood Type B is able to efficiently metabolize animal protein, but there are limitations that require careful dietary navigation. For cardiovascular health, Blood Type B needs to consume proteins that are high in the amino acid arginine, which regulates nitric oxide that helps arteries relax and open up. Blood Type B should minimize methionine-rich protein sources, which can increase homocysteine levels. Chicken, one of the most popular food choices, disagrees with Blood Type B, because of the lectin contained in the organ and muscle meat, which can interfere with fat metabolism. Turkey does not contain this lectin, and is an excellent alternative to chicken. Chicken is also one of the most methionine-rich foods in the American diet, and can lead to elevated homocysteine levels in some individuals. The leaner cuts of lamb and mutton should be a part of your diet. They help build muscle and active tissue mass, increasing your metabolic rate. Blood Type B nonsecretors should increase their weekly intake of meat and poultry.

BLOOD TYPE B: MEAT/POULTRY			
Portion: 4–6 oz (men); 2–5 oz (women and children)			
	African	Caucasian	Asian
Secretor	3–6	2–6	2–5
Non-Secretor	4–7	4–7	4–7
		Times per week	

SUPER BENEFICIAL	BENEFICIAL	NEUTRAL: Allowed Frequently	NEUTRAL: Allowed Infrequently	AVOID
Lamb	Goat	Beef		All commercially processed meats
Mutton	Rabbit	Buffalo		Bacon/Ham/ Pork
	Venison	Liver (calf)		Chicken
		Ostrich		Cornish hen
		Pheasant		Duck
		Turkey		Goose
		Veal		Grouse
				Guinea hen
				Heart (beef)
				Horse
				Partridge
				Quail
				Squab
				Squirrel

SUPER BENEFICIAL	BENEFICIAL	NEUTRAL: Allowed Frequently	NEUTRAL: Allowed Infrequently	AVOID
				Sweetbreads Turtle

Special Variants: *Non-Secretor* BENEFICIAL: liver (calf); NEUTRAL (Allowed Frequently): heart (beef), horse, squab, sweetbreads.

Fish/Seafood

Fish and seafood are an excellent source of protein for Blood Type B. Fish is a treasure trove of dense nutrients, able to build active tissue mass, particularly for non-secretors. Seafood can also be a good source of docosahexaenoic acid (DHA), a nutrient needed for proper nerve, tissue, and growth function. Finally, many ocean fish are rich in omega-3 fatty acids, which can keep the blood fluid and flowing easily. Omega-3 fatty acids decrease the risk of arrhythmias, which can lead to sudden cardiac death, decrease triglyceride levels, and decrease the growth rate of plaque in the arteries. Cod and mackerel are rich in the amino acid arginine, while also containing moderate amounts of the amino acid lysine. Some health authorities believe that a high lysine/arginine ratio in foods helps lower the incidence and severity of certain viral conditions.

BLOOD TYPE B: FISH/SEAFOOD			
Portion: 4–6 oz (men); 2–5 oz (women and children)			
	African	Caucasian	Asian
Secretor	4–5	3–5	3–5
Non-Secretor	4–5	4–5	4–5
	Times per week		

SUPER BENEFICIAL	BENEFICIAL	NEUTRAL: Allowed Frequently	NEUTRAL: Allowed Infrequently	AVOID
Cod	Caviar	Abalone	Herring	Anchovy
Halibut	(sturgeon)	Bluefish	(pickled/	Barracuda
Mackerel	Croaker	Bullhead	smoked)	Bass (all)
Sardine	Flounder	Carp	Salmon	Beluga
	Grouper	Catfish	(smoked)	Butterfish
	Haddock	Chub	Scallop	Clam
	Hake	Cusk		Conch
	Harvest	Drum		Crab
	fish	Gray sole		Crayfish
	Mahi-mahi	Halfmoon		Eel
	Monkfish	fish		Frog
	Perch	Herring		Lobster
	(ocean)	(fresh)		Mussels
	Pickerel	Mullet		Octopus
	Pike	Muskel-		Oysters
	Porgy	lunge		Pollock
	Salmon	Opaleye		Shrimp
	Shad	Orange		Snail (*Helix*
	Sole	roughy		*pomatia*/
	Sturgeon	Parrot fish		escargot)
		Perch		Trout (all)
		(silver/		Yellowtail
		white/		
		yellow)		
		Pompano		
		Red		
		snapper		
		Rosefish		
		Sailfish		
		Scrod		
		Scup		
		Shark		
		Smelt		
		Sole (gray)		

SUPER BENEFICIAL	BENEFICIAL	NEUTRAL: Allowed Frequently	NEUTRAL: Allowed Infrequently	AVOID
		Squid (calamari)		
		Sucker		
		Sunfish		
		Swordfish		
		Tilapia		
		Tilefish		
		Tuna		
		Weakfish		
		Whitefish		
		Whiting		

Special Variants: *Non-Secretor* BENEFICIAL: carp; NEUTRAL (Allowed Frequently): barracuda, butterfish, caviar (sturgeon), flounder, halibut, pike, salmon, snail (*Helix pomatia/escargot*), sole, yellowtail; AVOID: scallops.

Dairy/Eggs

Dairy products can be eaten by almost all Blood Type B secretors and to a lesser degree by non-secretors. Blood Type B can employ smart dairy choices to build active tissue mass, helping to increase metabolism. However, non-secretors should avoid eating too much cheese, as you are more sensitive to many of the microbial strains in aged cheeses. This is more common if you are of African ancestry, but the sensitivity can also be found in Caucasian and Asian populations. This caution holds particularly true if you suffer from recurrent sinus infections or colds, as dairy products are often mucus producers. Eggs are a good source of DHA (docosahexaenoic acid) for Blood Type B and can be an integral part of your protein requirement, helping to build active tissue mass. Try to find dairy products that are both hormone-free and organic.

BLOOD TYPE B: EGGS

Portion: 1 egg

	African	Caucasian	Asian
Secretor	3–4	3–4	3–4
Non-Secretor	5–6	5–6	5–6
		Times per week	

BLOOD TYPE B: MILK AND YOGURT

Portion: 4–6 oz (men); 2–5 oz (women and children)

	African	Caucasian	Asian
Secretor	3–5	3–4	3–4
Non-Secretor	1–3	2–4	1–3
		Times per week	

BLOOD TYPE B: CHEESE

Portion: 3 oz (men); 2 oz (women and children)

	African	Caucasian	Asian
Secretor	3–4	3–5	3–4
Non-Secretor	1–4	1–4	1–4
		Times per week	

SUPER BENEFICIAL	BENEFICIAL	NEUTRAL: Allowed Frequently	NEUTRAL: Allowed Infrequently	AVOID
Kefir	Cottage cheese	Camembert	Brie	American cheese
Yogurt	Farmer cheese	Casein	Butter	Blue cheese
	Feta	Cream cheese	Buttermilk	Egg (duck/ goose/ quail)
	Goat cheese	Edam	Cheddar	Ice cream
	Milk (cow/ goat)	Egg (chicken)	Colby	
	Mozzarella	Emmenthal	Half-and-half	
			Jarlsberg	
			Monterey Jack	

SUPER BENEFICIAL	BENEFICIAL	NEUTRAL: Allowed Frequently	NEUTRAL: Allowed Infrequently	AVOID
	Paneer Ricotta	Ghee (clarified butter) Gouda Gruyère Neufchâtel Parmesan Provolone Quark Sour cream	Muenster Sherbet Swiss cheese Whey	

Special Variants: *Non-Secretor* BENEFICIAL: ghee (clarified butter), whey; NEUTRAL (Allowed Frequently): cottage cheese, milk (cow); AVOID: Camembert, cheddar, Emmenthal, Jarlsberg, Monterey Jack, Muenster, Parmesan, provolone, Swiss cheeses.

Oils

Blood Type B does best on monounsaturated oils and oils rich in omega series fatty acids. Olive oil fits the bill in both regards. Constituents in olive oil, such as flavonoids, squalenes, and polyphenols, act as powerful antioxidants. Use it as your primary cooking oil.

Make it a point to avoid sesame, sunflower, and corn oils, which can contain immunoreactive proteins that impair Blood Type B digestion. These oils can interfere with metabolic activity.

BLOOD TYPE B: OILS			
Portion: 1 tblsp			
	African	Caucasian	Asian
Secretor	5–8	5–8	5–8
Non-Secretor	3–7	3–7	3–6
		Times per week	

SUPER BENEFICIAL	BENEFICIAL	NEUTRAL: Allowed Frequently	NEUTRAL: Allowed Infrequently	AVOID
Olive	Walnut	Almond	Wheat germ	Avocado
		Black currant seed		Borage seed
				Canola
		Cod liver		Castor
		Evening primrose		Coconut
				Corn
		Flax (linseed)		Cottonseed
				Peanut
				Safflower
				Sesame
				Soy
				Sunflower

Special Variants: *Non-Secretor* BENEFICIAL: black currant seed, flax (linseed) walnut.

Nuts and Seeds

Nuts and seeds can be an important secondary source of protein for Blood Type B. Black walnuts can aid bowel health and are known to have properties that improve blood sugar regulation and lower cholesterol. As with other aspects of the Blood Type B Diet plan, there are some idiosyncratic elements to the choice of seeds and nuts: Several, such as sunflower and sesame, have B-agglutinating lectins and should be avoided.

BLOOD TYPE B: NUTS AND SEEDS			
Portion: Whole (handful); Nut Butters (2 tblsp)			
	African	Caucasian	Asian
Secretor	4–7	4–7	4–7
Non-Secretor	5–7	5–7	5–7
		Times per week	

SUPER BENEFICIAL	BENEFICIAL	NEUTRAL: Allowed Frequently	NEUTRAL: Allowed Infrequently	AVOID
Walnut (black)		Almond	Litchi	Cashew
		Almond butter	Macadamia	Filbert (hazelnut)
		Beechnut	Pecan	Peanut
		Brazil		Peanut butter
		Butternut		Pignolia (pine nut)
		Chestnut		Pistachio
		Flax (linseed)		Poppy seed
		Hickory		Pumpkin seed
		Walnut (English)		Safflower seed
				Sesame butter (tahini)
				Sesame seed
				Sunflower butter
				Sunflower seed

Special Variants: *Non-Secretor* BENEFICIAL: walnut (English); NEUTRAL (Allowed Frequently): pumpkin seed.

Beans and Legumes

Blood Type B can do well on the proteins found in many beans and legumes, although this food category does contain more than a few beans with problematic lectins. Soy products should be de-emphasized, as they are rich in a class of enzymes that can interact negatively with the B antigen. Several beans, such as mung beans, contain B-agglutinating lectins and should be avoided. Northern beans are rich in the B vitamin folic acid

(90 mcg per cup), which helps the body to metabolize and clear homocysteine from the circulation.

BLOOD TYPE B: BEANS AND LEGUMES			
Portion: 1 cup (cooked)			
	African	Caucasian	Asian
Secretor	5–7	5–7	5–7
Non-Secretor	3–5	3–5	3–5
			Times per week

SUPER BENEFICIAL	BENEFICIAL	NEUTRAL: Allowed Frequently	NEUTRAL: Allowed Infrequently	AVOID
Fava (broad) bean Northern bean	Kidney bean Lima bean Navy bean	Bean (green/ snap/ string) Cannellini bean Copper bean Jicama bean Pea (green/ pod/ snow) Tamarind bean White bean	Soy bean	Adzuki bean Black bean Black-eyed pea Garbanzo (chickpea) Lentil (all) Miso Mung bean/ sprout Pinto bean Soy cheese Soy milk Tempeh Tofu

Special Variants: *Non-Secretor* NEUTRAL (Allowed Frequently): fava (broad) bean, kidney bean, lima bean, navy bean, northern bean, soy milk; AVOID: soy bean.

Grains and Starches

Grains present a series of problems for Blood Type B, especially in the area of insulin regulation. Non-secretors should be even more careful of their consumption of complex carbohydrates because of their insulin sensitivities. Corn lectin increases body fat for Blood Type B, as do corn by-products. Rye and buckwheat should also be avoided; these foods contain lectins capable of exerting an insulinlike effect on the body, resulting in a decrease of active tissue mass and an increase in body fat. Minimize or avoid whole-wheat products. The agglutinin in whole wheat is a key trigger for carbohydrate intolerance. However, this lectin can often be milled out of the grain, or destroyed by sprouting. Be careful with so-called sprouted breads, such as the "Ezekiel 4:9" breads. There are many varieties, and some contain Blood Type B avoids. Oatmeal is SUPER BENEFICIAL for Blood Type B secretors. Eating oatmeal can mitigate the damaging effects of high fat meals on the walls of the blood vessels, in a way very similar to vitamin E. Oats also have quite a bit of soluble fiber, which can exert mild cholesterol-lowering effects. Oats are also one of the best plant sources of the amino acid arginine, used in the body as a building block for nitric acid synthesis.

BLOOD TYPE B: GRAINS AND STARCHES			
Portion: ½ cup dry (grains or pastas); 1 muffin; 2 slices of bread			
	African	**Caucasian**	**Asian**
Secretor	5–7	5–9	5–9
Non-Secretor	3–5	3–5	3–5
		Times per week	

SUPER BENEFICIAL	BENEFICIAL	NEUTRAL: Allowed Frequently	NEUTRAL: Allowed Infrequently	AVOID
Oat bran	Essene bread (manna)	Barley	Rice flour	Amaranth
Oat flour		Quinoa	Soy flour/ products	Buckwheat
Oatmeal				Cornmeal

SUPER BENEFICIAL	BENEFICIAL	NEUTRAL: Allowed Frequently	NEUTRAL: Allowed Infrequently	AVOID
	Ezekiel 4:9 bread Millet Rice bran Rice cake Rice milk Spelt (whole)	Spelt flour/ products	Wheat (refined/ un- bleached) Wheat (semo- lina) Wheat (white flour)	Couscous Grits Kamut Popcorn Rice (wild) Rye Rye flour Soba noodles (100% buckwheat) Sorghum Tapioca Teff Wheat (whole) Wheat bran Wheat germ

Special Variants: *Non-Secretor* NEUTRAL (Allowed Frequently): amaranth, oat (all), rice (wild), sorghum, spelt (whole), tapioca; AVOID: soy flour/products, wheat (all).

Vegetables

Vegetables provide a rich source of antioxidants and fiber and also help to lower the production of toxins in the digestive tract. Many vegetables are rich in potassium, which helps to lower extracellular water in the body while raising the levels of intracellular water. Mushrooms (especially shiitake) are SUPER BENEFICIAL for Blood Type B. There is published evidence that mushrooms stimulate insulin production, which can help regulate fat metabolism. Blood Type B non-secretors can especially benefit from adding onions and garlic to their diets; they are rich in the amino acid citrulline, which can be used to manufacture nitric oxide. Although garlic and onions are only NEUTRAL for Type B secretors, all of the NEUTRAL or BENEFICIAL vegetables are of great benefit if you are trying to lose weight. Collards are rich in the B vitamin folic acid (64 mcg per ½ cup), which helps the body to metabolize and clear homocysteine from the circulation.

Tomatoes contain a lectin that reacts with the saliva and digestive juices of Blood Type B secretors, although it does not appear to react with non-secretors. Corn has B-agglutinating activity and should be avoided.

An item's value also applies to its juice, unless otherwise noted.

BLOOD TYPE B: VEGETABLES			
Portion: 1 cup, prepared (cooked or raw)			
	African	Caucasian	Asian
Secretor Super/ Beneficials	Unlimited	Unlimited	Unlimited
Secretor Neutrals	2–5	2–5	2–5
Non-Secretor Super/ Beneficials	Unlimited	Unlimited	Unlimited
Non-Secretor Neutrals	2–3	2–3	2–3
	Times per day		

SUPER BENEFICIAL	BENEFICIAL	NEUTRAL: Allowed Frequently	NEUTRAL: Allowed Infrequently	AVOID
Beet	Brussels	Alfalfa	Potato	Aloe
Beet	sprouts	sprouts		Artichoke
greens	Cabbage	Arugula		Corn
Broccoli	Cabbage	Asparagus		Olive (all)
Collards	(juice)*	Asparagus		Pumpkin
Kale	Carrot	pea		Radish/
Mushroom	Cauli-	Bamboo		sprouts
(shiitake)	flower	shoot		Rhubarb
Mustard	Eggplant	Bok choy		Tomato
greens	Parsnip			

SUPER BENEFICIAL	BENEFICIAL	NEUTRAL: Allowed Frequently	NEUTRAL: Allowed Infrequently	AVOID
	Peppers (all)	Carrot (juice)		
	Potato (sweet)	Celeriac		
		Celery		
	Yam	Chicory		
		Cucumber		
		Daikon radish		
		Dandelion		
		Endive		
		Escarole		
		Fennel		
		Fiddlehead fern		
		Garlic		
		Horse-radish		
		Kohlrabi		
		Leek		
		Lettuce (all)		
		Mushroom (abalone/ enoki/ maitake/ oyster/ porto-bello/ silver dollar/ straw/ tree ear)		
		Okra		
		Onion (all)		

SUPER BENEFICIAL	BENEFICIAL	NEUTRAL: Allowed Frequently	NEUTRAL: Allowed Infrequently	AVOID
		Oyster plant		
		Pickle (in brine or vinegar)		
		Poi		
		Radicchio		
		Rappini (broccoli rabe)		
		Rutabaga		
		Scallion		
		Seaweeds		
		Shallot		
		Spinach		
		Squash (all)		
		Swiss chard		
		Taro		
		Turnip		
		Water chestnut		
		Watercress		
		Yucca		
		Zucchini		

Special Variants: *Non-Secretor* SUPER BENEFICIAL: garlic, onion; BENEFICIAL: garlic, okra, onion (all); NEUTRAL (Allowed Frequently): artichoke, cabbage, eggplant, peppers (all), pumpkin, tomato; AVOID: potato.

*To obtain the benefits of cabbage juice, it must be consumed within one minute of juicing.

Fruits and Fruit Juices

A diet rich in proper fruits can help weight loss by tempering the effects of insulin. Also, fruits can help shift the balance of water in the body from high extracellular concentrations to high intracellular concentrations, thus preventing edema. Pineapples are rich in enzymes that help reduce inflammation and encourage proper water balance. Plums and prunes are high in the phytonutrients neochlorogenic and chlorogenic acid. These substances are classified as phenols, and their function as antioxidants has been well documented. Pineapple is rich in the B vitamin folic acid (58 mcg per cup), which helps the body to metabolize and clear homocysteine from the circulation. Cranberries, papaya, and elderberries are also good sources of folic acid. Watermelons are a good source of citrulline, ensuring proper nitric acid synthesis, while bananas are a very good source of pyridoxine (vitamin B_6), which, along with folic acid, can help control homocysteine levels.

Grapefruit juice is a well-documented culprit in many food-drug interactions. Grapefruit juice can inhibit the metabolism of certain heart and blood pressure drugs, including Nifedipine, Verapamil, and Lovastatin. Many readers have reported cautionary warnings of grapefruit's interaction appearing on Coumadin (warfarin prescriptions; blood thinners). There is no evidence in the medical literature to support this interaction. Grapefruit's effect on warfarin is insignificant.

An item's value also applies to its juice, unless otherwise noted.

BLOOD TYPE B: FRUITS AND FRUIT JUICES			
Portion: 1 cup			
	African	Caucasian	Asian
Secretor	2–4	3–5	3–5
Non-Secretor	2–3	2–3	2–3
		Times per day	

SUPER BENEFICIAL	BENEFICIAL	NEUTRAL: Allowed Frequently	NEUTRAL: Allowed Infrequently	AVOID
Banana	Grape	Apple	Apricot	Avocado
Cranberry	Plum	Blackberry	Asian pear	Bitter melon
Elderberry (dark blue/ purple)		Blueberry	Breadfruit	Coconut
		Boysen- berry	Cantaloupe	Persimmon
			Currant	Pomegranate

SUPER BENEFICIAL	BENEFICIAL	NEUTRAL: Allowed Frequently	NEUTRAL: Allowed Infrequently	AVOID
Papaya Pineapple Watermelon		Canang melon Casaba melon Cherry (all) Christmas melon Crenshaw melon Dewberry Gooseberry Grapefruit Guava Kiwi Kumquat Lemon Lime Loganberry Mango Mulberry Muskmelon Nectarine Orange Peach Pear Persian melon Prune Quince Raspberry Sago palm Spanish melon	Date Fig (fresh/ dried) Honeydew Plantain Raisin	Prickly pear Star fruit (carambola)

SUPER BENEFICIAL	BENEFICIAL	NEUTRAL: Allowed Frequently	NEUTRAL: Allowed Infrequently	AVOID
		Strawberry Tangerine Youngberry		

Special Variants: *Non-Secretor* BENEFICIAL: blackberry, blueberry, boysenberry, cherry, currant, fig (fresh/dried), guava, raspberry; NEUTRAL (Allowed Frequently): banana; AVOID: cantaloupe, honeydew.

Spices/Condiments/Sweeteners

Many spices have mild to moderate medicinal properties, often through their influence upon the balance of bacteria in the lower intestine, enabling the proper digestion and metabolism of foods. For Blood Type B, fenugreek is SUPER BENEFICIAL for its cardiovascular effects, which include lowering triglycerides. Turmeric is also SUPER BENEFICIAL because of a powerful chemical called curcumin. It has been shown to lower harmful cholesterol levels, to inhibit blood clotting by blocking prostaglandin production, and to help prevent or remedy arteriosclerosis. Ginger has profound effects on cardiovascular health, including preventing arteriosclerosis, lowering cholesterol levels, and preventing the oxidation of low-density lipoprotein (LDL).

Many common food additives, such as guar gum and carrageenan, should be avoided as they can enhance the effects of lectins found in other foods.

SUPER BENEFICIAL	BENEFICIAL	NEUTRAL: Allowed Frequently	NEUTRAL: Allowed Infrequently	AVOID
Fenugreek Ginger Turmeric	Horse-radish Molasses (black-strap)	Anise Apple pectin Basil	Agar Arrowroot Chocolate Fructose	Allspice Almond extract Aspartame

SUPER BENEFICIAL	BENEFICIAL	NEUTRAL: Allowed Frequently	NEUTRAL: Allowed Infrequently	AVOID
	Parsley	Bay leaf	Honey	Barley malt
	Pepper (cayenne)	Bergamot	Maple syrup	Carrageenan
		Caper	Mayon- naise	Cinnamon
		Caraway	Molasses	Cornstarch
		Cardamom	Pickles (all)	Corn syrup
		Carob	Rice syrup	Gelatin (ex- cept veg- sourced)
		Chervil	Sugar (brown/ white)	Guarana
		Chili powder	Tamari (wheat- free)	Gums (acacia/ Arabic/ guar)
		Chive	Vinegar (all)	Invert sugar
		Cilantro (coriander leaf)		Juniper
		Clove		Ketchup
		Coriander		Maltodextrin
		Cream of tartar		MSG
		Cumin		Pepper (black/ white)
		Dill		Soy sauce
		Garlic		Stevia
		Lecithin		Sucanat
		Mace		Tapioca
		Marjoram		
		Mint (all)		
		Mustard (dry)		
		Nutmeg		
		Oregano		
		Paprika		
		Pepper (pepper- corn/red flakes)		
		Rosemary		

SUPER BENEFICIAL	BENEFICIAL	NEUTRAL: Allowed Frequently	NEUTRAL: Allowed Infrequently	AVOID
		Saffron		
		Sage		
		Savory		
		Sea salt		
		Seaweeds		
		Senna		
		Tamarind		
		Tarragon		
		Thyme		
		Vanilla		
		Winter-green		
		Yeast (baker's/brewer's)		

Special Variants: *Non-Secretor* BENEFICIAL: oregano, yeast (brewer's); NEUTRAL (Allowed Frequently): stevia; AVOID: agar, fructose, pickle relish, sugar (brown/white).

Herbal Teas

Herbal teas can provide medicinal benefits, and several are SUPER BENEFICIAL for Blood Type B cardiovascular health. Ginseng helps reduce the effects of stress and improve overall cardiac health. Dandelion is rich in potassium and is a very mild diuretic. Ginger has profound effects on cardiovascular health, including preventing arteriosclerosis, lowering cholesterol levels, and preventing the oxidation of low-density lipoprotein (LDL).

SUPER BENEFICIAL	BENEFICIAL	NEUTRAL: Allowed Frequently	NEUTRAL: Allowed Infrequently	AVOID
Dandelion	Licorice root*	Alfalfa	Dong quai	Aloe
Ginger	Parsley	Burdock		Coltsfoot
Ginseng	Peppermint	Catnip		Corn silk
	Raspberry Leaf	Chamomile		Fenugreek
	Rosehip	Chickweed		Gentian
	Sage	Echinacea		Goldenseal
		Elder		Hops
		Hawthorn		Linden
		Horehound		Mullein
		Mulberry		Red clover
		Rosemary		Rhubarb
		Sarsaparilla		Shepherd's purse
		Senna		Skullcap
		Slippery elm		
		St. John's wort		
		Strawberry leaf		
		Thyme		
		Valerian		
		Vervain		
		White birch		
		White oak bark		
		Yarrow		
		Yellow dock		

Special Variants: None.

*Do not use if you have high blood pressure.

Miscellaneous Beverages

Blood Type B non-secretors may wish to have a glass of red wine two to four times a week. There are substantial cardiovascular benefits from moderate use. Secretors may have coffee, but try to limit your intake to one cup a day. Green tea is an excellent substitute for coffee, and helps prevent lipid oxidation. It can lower cholesterol by increasing the amount of a liver protein that helps to clear cholesterol from the blood.

SUPER BENEFICIAL	BENEFICIAL	NEUTRAL: Allowed Frequently	NEUTRAL: Allowed Infrequently	AVOID
Tea (green)		Wine (red/ white)	Beer Coffee (reg/ decaf) Tea, black (reg/ decaf)	Liquor Seltzer Soda (club) Soda (cola/ diet/misc.)

Special Variants: *Non-Secretor* BENEFICIAL: wine (red/white); NEUTRAL (Allowed Frequently): liquor, seltzer, soda (club); AVOID: coffee (reg/decaf), tea (black: reg/ decaf).

Supplements

THE BLOOD TYPE B Diet offers abundant quantities of important nutrients, such as protein and iron. It is important to get as many nutrients as possible from fresh foods and use supplements only to fill in the minor deficiencies in your diet. The following supplement protocols are designed for Blood Type B individuals who are suffering from cardiovascular disease or related conditions.

Note: If you are being treated for a cardiovascular or related condition, consult your doctor before taking any supplements.

Blood Type B: Cardiovascular Protection and Enhancement Protocol

Use this protocol for 4–8 weeks, then discontinue for 2 weeks and restart.

SUPPLEMENT	ACTION	DOSAGE
Coenzyme Q-10 (ubiquinone)	Improves coronary function	30–60 mg daily with meals
Magnesium	May help relax arteries, resulting in a slight decrease in blood pressure; mild blood-clot-inhibiting effects; produces mild improvement in angina	250–500 mg, once or twice daily
Vitamin C (food derived, from rosehip or acerola cherry)	May help protect against the oxidation of LDL cholesterol by neutralizing free radicals	100–200 mg daily
OPCs (oligomeric proanthocyandins)	Have antioxidant effects	100 mg daily
Fenugreek (*Trigonella foenum-graecum*)	Improves insulin production and reduces triglycerides	500 mg, twice daily

Blood Type B: Specific Cardiovascular Treatment Protocols

Use these protocols for 4–8 weeks, then discontinue for 1 week and restart. Protocols can be combined.

Cholesterol Control*		
SUPPLEMENT	ACTION	DOSAGE
Soluble fiber supplement	Mild cholesterol-lowering effects	3–5 grams daily

SUPPLEMENT	ACTION	DOSAGE
Green tea extracts	Reduce LDL cholesterol	1–2 capsules, twice daily. (Formula should contain a minimum of 150 mg of catechins, 150 mg of other tea anti-oxidants called polyphenols)
Pantethine (active vitamin B$_5$)	Lowers cholesterol	500 mg, twice daily

Stress Reduction Protocol

SUPPLEMENT	ACTION	DOSAGE
Dan Shen (*Salvia miltiorrhiza*)	Cardiovascular relaxant; stress modifier; promotes normal circulation in the body. (Note: should not be taken with pharmaceutical blood thinners, such as Coumadin or warfarin)	50 mg, once or twice daily
Spreading hogweed (*Boerhaavia diffusa*)	Acts as a stress modifier and a liver protector; lowers cortisol	50–150 mg, twice daily
Holy basil (*Ocimum sanctum*) leaf extract	Lowers cortisol	50 mg, twice daily

Angina Relief Adjunct*

SUPPLEMENT	ACTION	DOSAGE
Coenzyme Q-10 (ubiquinone)	Improves coronary function; reduces angina	30–60 mg daily with meals
L-arginine	Researchers have begun to use arginine in people with angina and congestive heart failure.	1000–2000 mg, twice daily

SUPPLEMENT	ACTION	DOSAGE
Jiaogulan (*Gynostemma pentaphyllum*)	Dramatically decreases the chances of a stroke by inhibiting blood platelets from sticking together, which prevents blood clots from forming. Also prevents artery clogging, reducing heart attack risk. By increasing nitric oxide, a chemical that relaxes blood vessel walls, it increases blood flow. It also reduces cholesterol by about 25%.	50–100 mg, twice daily

Hypertension Control*

SUPPLEMENT	ACTION	DOSAGE
Dandelion (*Taraxacum officinale*)	Mild diuretic, rich in electrolytes	150 mg, twice daily
L-arginine	Mild to moderate effects on high blood pressure; increases nitric oxide production, which relaxes artery walls	1000–2000 mg, twice daily
Cordyceps sinensis	Mild to moderate effects on arterial tension; good adaptogenic herb	100–250 mg, twice daily

Homocysteine Control*

SUPPLEMENT	ACTION	DOSAGE
Folic acid	Lowers homocysteine and builds blood	400 mcg, twice daily

SUPPLEMENT	ACTION	DOSAGE
Pyridoxine (vitamin B_6)	Works with folic acid to help metabolize homocysteine	50 mg, twice daily
Vitamin B_{12} (methylcobalamine)	Works with folic acid to help metabolize homocysteine	1000 mcg daily

*Check with your doctor before beginning this or any other nutritional protocol, especially if you are currently taking prescription medication.

The Exercise Component

FOR BLOOD TYPE B, stress regulation and overall fitness are achieved with a balance of moderate aerobic activity and mentally soothing, stress-reducing exercises. Below is a list of exercises that are recommended for Blood Type B.

EXERCISE	DURATION	FREQUENCY
Tennis	45–60 minutes	2–3 x week
Martial arts	30–60 minutes	2–3 x week
Cycling	45–60 minutes	2–3 x week
Hiking	30–60 minutes	2–3 x week
Golf (no cart!)	60–90 minutes	2–3 x week
Running or brisk walking	40–50 minutes	2–3 x week
Pilates	40–50 minutes	2–3 x week
Swimming	45 minutes	2–3 x week
Yoga	40–50 minutes	1–2 x week
T'ai Chi	40–50 minutes	1–2 x week

3 Steps to Effective Exercise

1. Warm up with stretching and flexibility moves before you start your aerobic exercise.
2. To achieve maximum cardiovascular benefits, work toward an elevated heart rate that is about 70 percent of your capacity. Once you reach the elevated rate, continue exercising to maintain that rate for twenty to thirty minutes. To calculate your maximum heart rate and performance level:
   - Subtract your age from 220.
   - Multiply the difference by .70 (or .60 if you are over age sixty). This is the high end of your performance.
   - Multiply the remainder by .50. This is the low end of your performance.
3. Finish each aerobic session with at least a five-minute cooldown of stretching and relaxation moves.

Getting Started: The First Month

IF YOU ARE NEW to the Blood Type Diet, the following guidelines will introduce you to the Blood Type B regimen over a period of one month. Follow these recommendations as closely as possible, using a journal to record your personal experiences with the diet. In addition to factors that are measurable in medical tests (EKG, cholesterol levels, blood pressure, cardiac stress tests), take the time to note changes in your energy levels, pain levels, sleep patterns, digestion, and overall well-being.

Week 1

Blood Type Diet and Supplements

- Eliminate your most harmful AVOID foods—chicken, corn, and buckwheat. The lectins in these foods can trigger inflammation.
- Avoid wheat if you are overweight or insulin-resistant.

Blood Type B Cardiovascular Diet Checklist

Eat small to moderate portions of high-quality, lean, organic ☐
meat (especially goat, lamb, and mutton) several times a week
for strength, energy, and digestive health. Meat should be prepared medium to rare for the best health effects. If you charbroil or cook meat well-done, use a marinade composed of
beneficial ingredients, such as cherry juice, spices, and herbs.

Include regular portions of richly oiled cold-water fish. Fish ☐
oils can improve cardiac health and contribute to lower cholesterol and triglyceride levels. They can also help counter inflammatory conditions and balance immune activity.

If you are not accustomed to eating dairy products, introduce ☐
them gradually, after you have been on the diet for Blood
Type B for several weeks. Begin with cultured dairy foods,
such as yogurt and kefir, which are more easily tolerated.

Eliminate wheat and wheat-based products from your diet. ☐
They are the gateway to metabolic syndrome and cardiovascular disease for your blood type.

Eat lots of BENEFICIAL fruits and vegetables. ☐

If you need a daily dose of caffeine, replace coffee with green ☐
tea. It isn't acidic and has substantially less caffeine than a cup
of coffee.

Use BENEFICIAL and NEUTRAL nuts and dried fruits for snacks. ☐

Avoid foods that are Type B red flags, especially chicken, ☐
corn, buckwheat, peanuts, lentils, and potatoes.

- Include your most important BENEFICIAL foods on a regular schedule throughout the week. For example, have lean red meat 5 times and omega-3-rich fish 3 to 4 times, with lots of BENEFICIAL vegetables and fruit.

- Incorporate at least 1 SUPER BENEFICIAL food into your daily diet. For example, have a handful of walnuts as a snack or eat yogurt mixed with berries for lunch.

- If you're a coffee drinker, begin to wean yourself by cutting your daily consumption in half, substituting green tea or a SUPER BENEFICIAL herbal tea.

Exercise Regimen

- Plan to exercise at least 4 days this week, for 45 minutes each day.

  2–3 days: aerobic activity

  1–2 days: yoga or T'ai Chi

- If you experience angina during exercise, consult with a physician. Angina is a warning sign that some of your heart muscle is not getting enough oxygen.

- If you are not accustomed to aerobic exercise, start slowly and gradually increase your duration and intensity of activity. The important factor is consistency. Just do it—as much as you're able.

- Use your journal to detail the time, activity, distance, and amount of weight. Note the number of repetitions for each exercise.

▪ WEEK 1 SUCCESS STRATEGY ▪
Fight Carbohydrate Cravings

If you crave any form of stimulants or carbohydrates, your serotonin levels are low, and your brain is demanding stimulants to raise your serotonin levels.

Try drinking some unsweetened cocoa powder in hot water or in a protein smoothie. Chocolate contains small amounts of serotonin, which explains why we feel so good when we eat it. Try a sip of vegetable glycerine between meals to cut down on your cravings. Avoid using the herbal serotonin supplements, such as 5HTP, on the market. The source material (griffonia seed) has a Type B–reactive lectin, which could be a problem.

Week 2

Blood Type Diet and Supplements

- Begin to eliminate the next level of AVOID foods—seeds, beans, and legumes—that have negative lectin activity.
- Eat at least 2 to 3 BENEFICIAL animal proteins every day—such as lamb, yogurt, or seafood.
- Initially, it is best to avoid foods listed as NEUTRAL: Allowed Infrequently.
- Continue to incorporate SUPER BENEFICIAL foods into your daily diet.
- If you're a coffee drinker, continue to cut your coffee intake, replacing it with green tea or SUPER BENEFICIAL herbal teas.

Exercise Regimen

- Continue to exercise at least 4 days this week, for 45 minutes each day.

  2–3 days: aerobic activity

  1–2 days: yoga or T'ai Chi

- If your work is sedentary, get in the habit of taking a couple of "movement" breaks during the day. Walk around the block or up and down stairs.

■ WEEK 2 SUCCESS STRATEGY ■
Think Yourself Healthy

Take advantage of Blood Type B's natural ability to relieve stress through meditation or guided imagery. I've never medicated Type B individuals who have high blood pressure without first teaching them some simple visualization techniques and sending them home to try them out for a few weeks. Those that did almost never required medication.

Here is a very simple visualization exercise to help control high blood pressure. Do this visualization two to four times daily for five to eight minutes.

Find a quiet place, and make yourself comfortable and re-laxed. Close your eyes and let your arms and hands lie limply at your sides or in your lap. Take a few deep breaths, inhaling through your nose and exhaling through your mouth, while imag-ining the red blood cells of your circulatory system coursing through your arteries and veins. See them slipping and sliding along the walls, which periodically open up like Venetian blinds to allow cells to move from the inside of the arteries out and from the outside in. Imagine the walls of your arteries relaxing and bending. Now expand the image and visualize your entire body. See the blood circulating from your heart to the arteries, to the capillaries, to the veins, then back to the lungs and heart.

Week 3

Blood Type Diet and Supplements

- When you plan your meals for week 3, choose BENEFICIAL foods to replace NEUTRAL foods whenever possible. For example, choose lamb over beef, or blueberries over an apple.
- Eliminate all remaining AVOID foods.
- Liberally incorporate SUPER BENEFICIAL foods into your daily diet.

Exercise Regimen

- Continue to exercise at least 4 days this week, for 45 minutes each day.

  2–3 days: aerobic activity

  1–2 days: yoga or T'ai Chi

■ **WEEK 3 SUCCESS STRATEGY** ■
The B Health Cocktail

Extra arginine and folic acid are beneficial to your health. You may want to drink this specially formulated Membrane Fluidizer Cardio Cocktail every day.

1 tablespoon olive oil
1 tablespoon high quality lecithin granules
(sources other than soy would be best)
6–8 ounces of a combination of papaya, banana,
watermelon, and/or pineapple juice
The juice of ½" to 1" piece fresh ginger (pungent!)

Combine, shake well, and drink.

Week 4

Blood Type Diet and Supplements

- Continue at the week 3 level, focusing on BENEFICIAL and SUPER BENEFICIAL foods.
- Evaluate the first 4 weeks and make adjustments.

Exercise Regimen

- Continue at the week 3 level.
- Review your progress, noting in your journal improvements in strength and flexibility. Determine which exercise regimen has worked for you, including time of day, setting, and activity level.

■ WEEK 4 SUCCESS STRATEGY ■
Sleep Tight

High cortisol levels can disrupt your sleep cycle. You may have to work harder to stay energized. Try to establish a regular sleep schedule and adhere to it as closely as possible. When you have a normal sleep-wake rhythm, it reduces cortisol levels. During the day, schedule at least two breaks of 20 minutes each for complete relaxation. Combat sleep disturbances with regular exercise and a relaxing pre-bedtime routine. A light snack before bedtime will help raise your blood sugar levels and improve sleep. If these strategies don't work, ask your doctor about the following supplements:

Methylcobalamin (active vitamin B$_{12}$): 1 to 3 mg per day taken in the morning. This vitamin enables deep sleep and helps you wake feeling more rested. Methylcobalamin also increases the action of folic acid in lowering homocysteine.

A Final Word

IN SUMMARY, the secret to fighting cardiovascular disease with the Blood Type B Diet involves:

1. Increasing active tissue mass (calorie-burning tissue) by switching to a more animal protein–based diet.
2. Minimizing consumption of the insulin-mimicking lectins most abundant in grains such as wheat and corn, which can contribute to metabolic syndrome, a precursor to heart disease.
3. Increasing circulatory efficiency and reducing stress by adopting an exercise program that combines vigorous routines with calming activities.
4. Using supplements intelligently to block the effect of insulin-mimicking lectins, provide antioxidant support, enhance nitric oxide production, and help lower homocysteine.

Blood Type
AB

BLOOD TYPE AB DIET OUTCOME: MULTIPLE BENEFITS
"Because of a diagnosis of atrial fibrillation and elevated triglycerides, at 200 pounds (I'm 5'7"), I undertook the Blood Type Diet in earnest. I have lost 25 pounds in three months. As a side benefit, my strength, endurance, and digestion are better than they have been in years."

BLOOD TYPE AB DIET OUTCOME: THE ANSWER TO HER PRAYERS
"I'm now entering my second month on the Blood Type Diet, and I feel so much better. I used to sleep about fifteen hours a day, and now I'm down to eight hours. Because of that, I've lost a lot of weight. Even my family is eating much better. There is less candy in the house, and more fruit and veggies. This has been the answer to my prayers."

Self-reported outcomes from the Blood Type Diet Web site (www.dadamo.com).

BLOOD TYPE AB HAS A SOMEWHAT MIXED PROFILE WHEN it comes to cardiovascular disease. Overall, you share Blood Type A's relatively high risk for cardiovascular disease, although the B antigen conveys some help in preventing and fighting it. A number of studies show that Blood Types A and AB are more likely to be at risk of heart disease and death by virtue of elevated cholesterol. The underlying reason for this tendency is your difficulty breaking down dietary fats due to lower levels of the enzyme responsible for this function, intestinal alkaline phosphatase. Blood Type AB is somewhat better able to break down fat than Blood Type A, but you need to limit the amount of animal protein you consume.

Like Blood Type A, you also have high levels of the blood clotting factor, factor VIII, which has been linked to coronary artery disease. Greater blood viscosity (thickness) increases the potential for developing arterial blood clots.

Also similar to Blood Type A, Blood Type AB tends to have higher levels of binding sites (selectins) that the white blood cells of the immune system use to attach to vessel walls as a prelude to moving into the tissues. When this process is out of control, the delicate lining of the blood vessels can become damaged, thus attracting platelets (specialized clotting cells), and eventually resulting in calcification and narrowing of the opening, or lumen.

Another potential cardiovascular challenge for Blood Type AB involves the ineffective regulation of nitric oxide, a chemical released by the cells lining the artery walls. Nitric oxide allows blood vessels to relax and open up. Arginine-rich foods are a great way to enhance nitric oxide production.

Because you also share some B-specific characteristics, you must also be careful to avoid certain antimetabolic lectins that react with the B antigen. Overall, the best guidelines for Blood Type AB involve a combination of the best of the A and B worlds.

Blood Type AB

TOP TWELVE HEART-HEALTHY FOODS

1. Soy foods
2. Richly oiled cold-water fish
3. Cultured dairy foods (yogurt, kefir)
4. Olive oil
5. Walnuts
6. Maitake mushrooms
7. Leafy green vegetables
8. Cherries, gooseberries, loganberries
9. Pineapple
10. Garlic
11. Ginger
12. Green tea

Blood Type AB: The Foods

THE BLOOD TYPE AB Cardiovascular Diet is specifically adapted for the prevention and management of cardiovascular disease. A new category, **Super Beneficial**, highlights powerful disease-fighting foods for Blood Type AB. The **Neutral** category has also been adjusted to de-emphasize foods that are less advantageous for you. Foods designated **Neutral: Allowed Infrequently** should be minimized or avoided entirely.

Food Values

SUPER BENEFICIAL	Foods that are known to have specific disease-fighting qualities for your blood type.
BENEFICIAL	Foods with components that enhance the metabolic, immune, or structural health of you blood type.

NEUTRAL Allowed frequently	Foods that normally have no direct blood type effect but supply a variety of nutrients necessary for a healthful diet.
NEUTRAL Allowed infrequently	Foods that normally have no blood type effect but may impede your progress when consumed regularly.
AVOID	Foods with components that are harmful to your blood type.

Your secretor status can influence your ability to fully digest and metabolize certain foods, so various adjustments in the values are made for non-secretors. If you do not know your secretor type, the odds are that you can safely use the "secretor" values, since the majority of the population (approximately 80 percent) are secretors. However, I urge you to get tested, since the variations are important for non-secretors who want to maximize the effectiveness of the Blood Type Diet.

The food charts are divided into three sections. The top of the chart suggests the average portion size and quantity per week or day, according to secretor status. These recommendations do *not* apply to the category **Neutral: Allowed Infrequently**; those foods should be eaten rarely, if at all. The charts also indicate differences in frequency for some foods, based on ethnic heritage. It has been my experience that this factor has an impact upon the individual's ability to fully digest certain foods. For the purposes of blood type food choices, persons of Hispanic heritage should follow the recommendations for Caucasians; North American Native peoples should follow the recommendations for Asians.

The middle section of the chart gives the food values. The bottom section lists variants based on secretor status.

For your convenience, we have included a number of product names (Ezekiel 4:9 bread, Worcestershire sauce, etc.). However, keep in mind that commercial formulations vary among brands and regions. Even though a product may be listed as acceptable for you, always check its ingredients; do not use products that contain **Avoid** ingredients for your blood type. Of course, you may choose to make your own version of commercial products, such as bread and mayonnaise, using ingredients that suit your blood type. There are hundreds of delicious recipes for every blood type available on our Web site (www.dadamo. com), and in the book *Cook Right 4 Your Type: The Practical Kitchen Companion to* Eat Right 4 Your Type.

Meat/Poultry

Blood Type AB is a bit more adapted to animal-based proteins than Blood Type A, mainly because of the B gene's effects on fat absorption. However, you need to limit your consumption and beware of elevated cholesterol. Excessive consumption of animal protein can aggravate the Blood Type AB tendency toward high LDL cholesterol, as well as accelerated blood clotting, which can cause arterial damage.

Chicken, one of the most popular food choices, disagrees with Blood Type AB, because of the lectin contained in the organ and muscle meat, which can interfere with fat metabolism. Turkey does not contain this lectin and is an excellent alternative to chicken. Chicken is also one of the most methionine-rich foods in the American diet, and can lead to elevated homocysteine levels in some individuals.

Choose only the highest-quality (preferably grass-fed) chemical-, antibiotic-, and pesticide-free low-fat meats and poultry.

BLOOD TYPE AB: MEATS/POULTRY			
Portion: 4–6 oz (men); 2–5 oz (women and children)			
	African	Caucasian	Asian
Secretor	2–5	1–5	1–5
Non-Secretor	3–5	2–5	2–5
		Times per week	

SUPER BENEFICIAL	BENEFICIAL	NEUTRAL: Allowed Frequently	NEUTRAL: Allowed Infrequently	AVOID
	Lamb	Goat	Liver (calf)	All commercially processed meats
	Mutton	Ostrich		
	Rabbit	Pheasant		
	Turkey			Bacon/Ham/ Pork
				Beef
				Buffalo
				Chicken
				Cornish hen
				Duck
				Goose
				Grouse
				Guinea hen
				Heart (beef)
				Partridge
				Quail
				Squab
				Squirrel
				Sweetbreads
				Turtle
				Veal
				Venison

Special Variants: *Non-Secretor* NEUTRAL (Allowed Frequently): quail, venison.

Fish/Seafood

Fish and seafood are an excellent source of protein for Blood Type AB. Fish is a treasure trove of dense nutrients, able to build active tissue mass, particularly for non-secretors. Seafood can also be a good source of docosahexaenoic acid (DHA), a nutrient needed for proper nerve, tissue, and growth function. Fish are also a good source of selenium, a nutrient essential to controlling arterial inflammation via its effects on selectins. Cod and mackerel are also good sources of arginine, an amino acid that helps form the artery-relaxing molecule nitric oxide. Finally, many ocean fish are rich in omega-3 fatty acids, which can keep the blood fluid flowing easily. Omega-3 fatty acids decrease the risk of arrhythmias (which can lead to sudden cardiac death), lower triglyceride levels, and decrease the growth rate of plaque in the arteries.

BLOOD TYPE AB: FISH/SEAFOOD			
Portion: 4–6 oz (men); 2–5 oz (women and children)			
	African	Caucasian	Asian
Secretor	4–6	3–5	3–5
Non-Secretor	4–7	4–6	4–6
			Times per week

SUPER BENEFICIAL	BENEFICIAL	NEUTRAL: Allowed Frequently	NEUTRAL: Allowed Infrequently	AVOID
Cod	Grouper	Abalone	Caviar	Anchovy
Mackerel	Mahi-mahi	Bluefish	(sturgeon)	Barracuda
Red snapper	Monkfish	Bullhead	Mussels	Bass (all)
Salmon	Pickerel	Butterfish	Scallop	Beluga
Sardine	Pike	Carp	Squid	Clam
	Porgy	Catfish	(calamari)	Conch
	Sailfish	Chub	Whitefish	Crab
	Shad	Croaker		Eel
	Snail (Helix pomatia/ escargot)	Cusk		Flounder
	Sturgeon	Drum		Frog
	Tuna	Halfmoon fish		Gray sole
		Harvest fish		Haddock
		Herring (fresh)		Hake
		Mullet		Halibut
				Herring (pickled/ smoked)

SUPER BENEFICIAL	BENEFICIAL	NEUTRAL: Allowed Frequently	NEUTRAL: Allowed Infrequently	AVOID
		Muskel-lunge		Lobster
		Opaleye		Octopus
		Orange roughy		Oysters
		Parrot fish		Salmon (smoked)
		Perch (all)		Salmon roe
		Pollock		Shrimp
		Pompano		Sole
		Rosefish		Trout (all)
		Scrod		Whiting
		Scup		Yellowtail
		Shark		
		Smelt		
		Sucker		
		Sunfish		
		Swordfish		
		Tilapia		
		Tilefish		
		Tuna		
		Weakfish		

Special Variants: *Non-Secretor* BENEFICIAL: herring (fresh); NEUTRAL (Allowed Frequently): trout (all).

Dairy/Eggs

Dairy products can be used with discretion by many Blood Type AB individuals, especially secretors. Eggs, a good source of DHA (docosahexaeonic acid), as is fish, can complement the protein profile for your blood type, helping to build active tissue mass. Most dairy products are rich in arginine and the amino acid lysine. Some health authorities believe that a high lysine/arginine ratio in foods helps lower the incidence and severity of certain viral conditions. If you are of African ancestry, you may need to minimize noncultured forms of dairy, such as milk.

BLOOD TYPE AB: EGGS			
Portion: 1 egg			
	African	**Caucasian**	**Asian**
Secretor	2–5	3–4	3–4
Non-Secretor	3–6	3–6	3–6
		Times per week	

BLOOD TYPE AB: MILK AND YOGURT			
Portion: 4–6 oz (men); 2–5 oz (women and children)			
	African	**Caucasian**	**Asian**
Secretor	2–6	3–6	1–6
Non-Secretor	0–3	0–4	0–3
		Times per week	

BLOOD TYPE AB: CHEESE			
Portion: 3 oz (men); 2 oz (women and children)			
	African	**Caucasian**	**Asian**
Secretor	2–3	3–4	3–4
Non-Secretor	0	0–1	0
		Times per week	

SUPER BENEFICIAL	BENEFICIAL	NEUTRAL: Allowed Frequently	NEUTRAL: Allowed Infrequently	AVOID
Kefir	Cottage	Casein	Cheddar	American
Milk (goat)	cheese	Cream	Colby	cheese
Yogurt	Egg	cheese	Emmenthal	Blue cheese
	(chicken)	Edam	Milk (cow)	Brie
				Butter

SUPER BENEFICIAL	BENEFICIAL	NEUTRAL: Allowed Frequently	NEUTRAL: Allowed Infrequently	AVOID
	Farmer cheese Feta Goat cheese Mozzarella Ricotta Sour cream	Egg (goose/ quail) Ghee (clarified butter) Gouda Gruyère Jarlsberg Muenster Neufchâtel Paneer Quark String cheese Whey	Monterey Jack Sherbet Swiss cheese	Buttermilk Camembert Egg (duck) Half-and-half Ice cream Parmesan Provolone

Special Variants: *Non-Secretor* BENEFICIAL: ghee (clarified butter); NEUTRAL (Allowed Frequently): goat cheese, yogurt; AVOID: Emmenthal, Swiss cheese.

Oils

Blood Type AB does best on monounsaturated oils and oils rich in omega series fatty acids. Olive oil fits the bill in both regards. Constituents in olive oil, such as flavonoids, squalenes, and polyphenols, act as powerful antioxidants. Use it as your primary cooking oil.

Make it a point to avoid sesame, sunflower, and corn oils, which can contain immunoreactive proteins that impair Blood Type AB digestion. These oils can interfere with metabolic activity.

BLOOD TYPE AB: OILS			
Portion: 1 tblsp			
	African	**Caucasian**	**Asian**
Secretor	4–7	5–8	5–7
Non-Secretor	3–6	3–6	3–6
		Times per week	

SUPER BENEFICIAL	BENEFICIAL	NEUTRAL: Allowed Frequently	NEUTRAL: Allowed Infrequently	AVOID
Olive	Walnut	Almond	Wheat germ	Avocado
		Black currant seed		Coconut
		Borage seed		Corn
		Canola		Cottonseed
		Castor		Safflower
		Cod liver		Sesame
		Evening primrose		Sunflower
		Flax (linseed)		
		Peanut		
		Soy		
Special Variants: None.				

Nuts and Seeds

Nuts and seeds are a good secondary protein source for Blood Type AB. Several nuts, such as walnuts, can help lower toxic concentrations in the intestine and are also known to improve blood sugar regulation and lower cholesterol. Peanuts are high in arginine, which can benefit the arteries. Walnuts are a great source of selenium, an antioxidant known to block arterial inflammation, one of the first stages of arteriosclerosis.

BLOOD TYPE AB: NUTS AND SEEDS			
Portion: Whole (handful); Nut Butters (2 tblsp)			
	African	**Caucasian**	**Asian**
Secretor	5–10	5–10	5–9
Non-Secretor	4–8	4–9	5–9
		Times per week	

SUPER BENEFICIAL	BENEFICIAL	NEUTRAL: Allowed Frequently	NEUTRAL: Allowed Infrequently	AVOID
Peanut	Chestnut	Almond	Brazil nut	Filbert
Peanut butter		Almond butter	Cashew	(hazelnut)
Walnut (black/ English)		Almond cheese	Cashew butter	Poppy seed
		Almond milk	Macadamia	Pumpkin seed
		Beechnut	Pecan	Sesame butter (tahini)
		Butternut	Pecan butter	Sesame seed
		Flax (linseed)	Pistachio	Sunflower butter
		Hickory	Safflower seed	Sunflower seed
		Litchi		
		Pignolia (pine nut)		

Special Variants: *Non-Secretor* NEUTRAL (Allowed Frequently): peanut, peanut butter; AVOID: Brazil nut, cashew, cashew butter, pistachio.

Beans and Legumes

Blood Type AB does well on proteins found in many beans and legumes, although this food category contains more than a few beans with problematic A- or B-specific lectins. In general, this category is only marginally sufficient to build active tissue mass in Blood Type AB, particularly non-secretors. In particular, Blood Type AB does well on soy foods, which not only have cardiovascular benefits (soy isoflavones are effective blockers of selectin activity, a marker of blood vessel inflammation) but also are essential to healthy immune system function for Blood Type AB. A number of studies have shown that the regular consumption of soy protein significantly reduces LDL cholesterol, especially for individuals with extremely high levels (over 355 mg/dL).

BLOOD TYPE AB: BEANS AND LEGUMES			
Portion: 1 cup (cooked)			
	African	Caucasian	Asian
Secretor	3–6	3–6	4–6
Non-Secretor	2–5	2–5	3–6
			Times per week

SUPER BENEFICIAL	BENEFICIAL	NEUTRAL: Allowed Frequently	NEUTRAL: Allowed Infrequently	AVOID
Miso	Lentil	Bean	Jicama	Adzuki bean
Soy bean	(green)	(green/	bean	Black bean
Tempeh	Navy bean	snap/		Black-eyed
Tofu	Pinto bean	string)		pea
		Cannellini		Fava (broad)
		bean		bean
		Copper		Garbanzo
		bean		(chickpea)
		Lentil		Kidney bean
		(domestic/		Lima bean
		red)		Mung bean/
		Northern		sprout
		bean		
		Pea (green/		
		pod/		
		snow)		
		Soy cheese		
		Soy milk		

SUPER BENEFICIAL	BENEFICIAL	NEUTRAL: Allowed Frequently	NEUTRAL: Allowed Infrequently	AVOID
		Tamarind bean White bean		

Special Variants: *Non-Secretor* NEUTRAL (Allowed Frequently): fava (broad) bean, miso, navy bean, soy bean, tempeh, tofu; AVOID; jicama bean, soy cheese, soy milk.

Grains and Starches

Blood Type AB secretors have many choices of grains, though only oats and soy offer any SUPER BENEFICIAL effects, mostly because they are an easily available form of soluble fiber (oats) or help block arterial inflammation (soy). Non-secretors, however, should limit their consumption of wheat and corn products. These foods contain lectins capable of exerting an antimetabolic effect on your body, lowering active tissue mass and increasing total body fat. However, the lectin in wheat can often be milled out of the grain, or destroyed by sprouting. Be care-

BLOOD TYPE AB: GRAINS AND STARCHES			
Portion: ½ cup dry (grains or pastas); 1 muffin; 2 slices of bread			
	African	Caucasian	Asian
Secretor	6–8	6–9	6–10
Non-Secretor	4–6	5–7	6–8
			Times per week

SUPER BENEFICIAL	BENEFICIAL	NEUTRAL: Allowed Frequently	NEUTRAL: Allowed Infrequently	AVOID
Oat bran Oat flour Oatmeal	Amaranth Essene bread (manna)	Barley Couscous Quinoa	Wheat (semolina) Wheat (whole)	Buckwheat Cornmeal Grits Kamut

SUPER BENEFICIAL	BENEFICIAL	NEUTRAL: Allowed Frequently	NEUTRAL: Allowed Infrequently	AVOID
Soy flour/ products	Ezekiel 4:9 bread	Spelt flour/ products	Wheat bran	Popcorn
	Millet		Wheat germ	Soba noodles (100% buck- wheat)
	Rice (whole)			
	Rice (wild)			Sorghum
	Rice bran			Tapioca
	Rice cake			Teff
	Rye (whole)			Wheat (refined/ un- bleached)
	Rye flour/ products			
	Spelt (whole)			Wheat (white flour)

Special Variants: *Non-Secretor* NEUTRAL (Allowed Frequently): Ezekiel 4:9 bread, spelt (whole); AVOID: soy flour/products, wheat (semolina), wheat germ, wheat (whole).

ful with so-called sprouted breads, such as the "Ezekiel 4:9" breads. There are many varieties, and some contain Blood Type AB avoids.

Vegetables

Vegetables provide a rich source of antioxidants and fiber and also help to lower the production of toxins in the digestive tract. Many vegetables are rich in potassium, which helps to lower extracellular water in the body while raising the levels of intracellular water. This can help relieve the load on the heart and increase cardiac output. Collards, a SUPER BENEFICIAL for Blood Type AB, are rich in the B vitamin folic acid (64 mcg per ½ cup), which helps the body to metabolize and clear homocysteine from the circulation. Garlic is SUPER BENEFI-CIAL for Blood Type AB because of its ability to reduce excess blood-clotting factors and because it is a good source of the amino acid citrulline, a potential precursor to nitric oxide metabolism. All of the neutral or beneficial vegetables are of great benefit to Blood Type AB, if you are trying to lose weight.

An item's value also applies to its juice, unless otherwise noted.

BLOOD TYPE AB: VEGETABLES			
Portion: 1 cup, prepared (cooked or raw)			
	African	**Caucasian**	**Asian**
Secretor Super/ Beneficials	Unlimited	Unlimited	Unlimited
Secretor Neutrals	2–5	2–5	2–5
Non-Secretor Super/ Beneficials	Unlimited	Unlimited	Unlimited
Non-Secretor Neutrals	2–3	2–3	2–3
		Times per day	

SUPER BENEFICIAL	BENEFICIAL	NEUTRAL: Allowed Frequently	NEUTRAL: Allowed Infrequently	AVOID
Beet	Alfalfa	Arugula	Carrot	Aloe
Beet greens	sprouts	Asparagus	Daikon radish	Artichoke
Broccoli	Cabbage (juice)*	Asparagus pea	Olive (Greek/ green/ Spanish)	Corn
Collards	Carrot (juice)	Bamboo shoot		Mushroom (abalone/ shiitake)
Garlic	Cauli- flower	Bok choy	Poi	Olive (black)
Kale	Celery	Brussels sprouts	Potato	Peppers (all)
Mustard greens	Cucumber	Cabbage	Pumpkin	Pickle (all)
	Dandelion	Celeriac	Taro	Radish/ sprouts
	Eggplant	Chicory		Rhubarb
	Mushroom (maitake)	Cucumber (juice)*		
	Parsnip	Endive		
	Potato (sweet)	Escarole		
		Fennel		

SUPER BENEFICIAL	BENEFICIAL	NEUTRAL: Allowed Frequently	NEUTRAL: Allowed Infrequently	AVOID
	Yam	Fiddlehead fern		
		Horse-radish		
		Kohlrabi		
		Leek		
		Lettuce (all)		
		Mushroom (enoki/ oyster/ porto-bello/ silver dollar/ straw/ tree ear)		
		Okra		
		Onion (all)		
		Oyster plant		
		Radicchio		
		Rappini (broccoli rabe)		
		Rutabaga		
		Scallion		
		Seaweeds		
		Shallot		
		Spinach		
		Squash (all)		
		Swiss chard		
		Tomato		
		Turnip		

SUPER BENEFICIAL	BENEFICIAL	NEUTRAL: Allowed Frequently	NEUTRAL: Allowed Infrequently	AVOID
		Water chestnut Watercress Yucca Zucchini		

Special Variants: *Non-Secretor* BENEFICIAL: tomato; NEUTRAL (Allowed Frequently): beet; AVOID: poi, taro.

*To obtain the benefits of cabbage and cucumber juices, they must be consumed within one minute of juicing.

Fruits and Fruit Juices

A diet rich in proper fruits can promote weight loss by tempering the effects of insulin. Also, fruits can help shift the balance of water in the body from high extracellular concentrations to high intracellular concentrations, lessening the stress on the heart. Pineapple is rich in enzymes that help reduce inflammation and encourage proper water balance. Pineapple is also a good source of the B vitamin folic acid (58 mcg per cup), which helps the body to metabolize and clear homocysteine from the circulation. Cranberries and many other berries are also good sources of folic acid. Watermelon is a good source of citrulline, insuring proper nitric acid synthesis. Lemon is a natural blood thinner.

Grapefruit juice is a well-documented culprit in many food-drug interactions. Grapefruit juice can inhibit the metabolism of certain heart and blood pressure drugs, including Nifedipine, Verapamil, and Lovastatin. Many readers have reported cautionary warnings of grapefruit's interaction appearing on Coumadin (warfarin prescriptions; blood thinners). There is no evidence in the medical literature to support this interaction. Grapefruit's effect on warfarin is insignificant.

If you are a non-secretor, you'll need to watch your intake of high glucose-containing fruits, especially if you are sensitive to sugar.

An item's value also applies to its juices, unless otherwise noted.

BLOOD TYPE AB: FRUITS AND FRUIT JUICES

Portion: 1 cup

	African	Caucasian	Asian
Secretor	3–4	3–6	3–5
Non-Secretor	1–3	2–3	3–4
		Times per day	

SUPER BENEFICIAL	BENEFICIAL	NEUTRAL: Allowed Frequently	NEUTRAL: Allowed Infrequently	AVOID
Cherry	Fig (fresh/	Apple	Apricot	Avocado
Cranberry	dried)	Blackberry	Asian pear	Banana
Gooseberry	Grape (all)	Blueberry	Breadfruit	Bitter melon
Lemon	Grapefruit	Boysen-	Canang	Coconut
Loganberry	Kiwi	berry	melon	Dewberry
Pineapple	Plum	Elderberry	Cantaloupe	Guava
Watermelon		(dark	Casaba	Mango
		blue/	melon	Orange
		purple)	Christmas	Persimmon
		Grapefruit	melon	Pomegranate
		(juice)*	Crenshaw	Prickly pear
		Kumquat	melon	Quince
		Lime	Currant	Sago palm
		Mulberry	Date	Star fruit
		Muskmelon	Honeydew	(carambola)
		Nectarine	Prune	
		Papaya	Raisin	
		Peach	Tangerine	
		Pear		
		Persian		
		melon		
		Pineapple		
		(juice)		
		Plantain		
		Raspberry		
		Spanish		
		melon		

SUPER BENEFICIAL	BENEFICIAL	NEUTRAL: Allowed Frequently	NEUTRAL: Allowed Infrequently	AVOID
		Strawberry Young-berry		

Special Variants: *Non-Secretor* BENEFICIAL: blackberry, blueberry, elderberry, lime; NEUTRAL (Allowed Frequently): banana; AVOID: cantaloupe, honeydew, prune, tangerine.

Spices/Condiments/Sweeteners

Many spices have mild to moderate medicinal properties, often by influencing the levels of bacteria in the lower colon. Turmeric is also SUPER BENEFICIAL because of a powerful chemical called curcumin. Curcumin has been shown to lower harmful cholesterol levels, inhibit blood clotting by blocking prostaglandin production, and to help prevent or remedy arteriosclerosis, thus playing a significant role in the prevention of heart and arterial disease. Ginger has profound effects on cardiovascular health, including preventing arteriosclerosis, lowering cholesterol levels, preventing the oxidation of low-density lipoprotein (LDL), and reducing blood clotting. Coriander seeds have been shown to enhance the synthesis of bile acid by the liver, lowering overall cholesterol. They have also been shown to increase HDL ("good") cholesterol. Garlic has mild to moderate effects on cholesterol. Parsley is an excellent source of potassium, which is important in lowering blood pressure. It also supplies folic acid, which helps prevent cardiovascular disease. Always use fresh parsley, as the antioxidants are destroyed by drying.

Many common food additives, such as guar gum and carrageenan, should be avoided as they can enhance the effects of lectins found in other foods.

SUPER BENEFICIAL	BENEFICIAL	NEUTRAL: Allowed Frequently	NEUTRAL: Allowed Infrequently	AVOID
Coriander seeds	Horse-radish	Basil	Agar	Allspice
Garlic	Molasses (black-strap)	Bay leaf	Apple pectin	Almond extract
Ginger		Bergamot	Arrowroot	Anise
Oregano		Caraway	Chocolate	Aspartame
Parsley		Cardamom	Honey	Barley malt
Turmeric		Carob	Maple syrup	Carrageenan
		Chervil	Mayon-naise	Cornstarch
		Chili powder	Molasses	Corn syrup
		Chive	Rice syrup	Dextrose
		Cilantro (corian-der leaf)	Senna	Fructose
		Cinnamon	Soy sauce	Gelatin (ex-cept veg-sourced)
		Clove	Sugar (brown/white)	Guarana
		Cream of tartar		Gums (acacia/Arabic/guar)
		Cumin		Invert sugar
		Dill		Ketchup
		Juniper		Maltodextrin
		Licorice root*		MSG
		Mace		Pepper (black/white)
		Marjoram		Pepper (cayenne)
		Mint (all)		
		Mustard (dry)		
		Nutmeg		
		Paprika		
		Rosemary		
		Saffron		
		Sage		

SUPER BENEFICIAL	BENEFICIAL	NEUTRAL: Allowed Frequently	NEUTRAL: Allowed Infrequently	AVOID
		Savory		Pepper (peppercorn/ red flakes)
		Sea salt		Pickles (all)
		Seaweeds		Sucanat
		Stevia		Tapioca
		Tamari (wheat-free)		Vinegar (all)
		Tamarind		Worcester-shire sauce
		Tarragon		
		Thyme		
		Vanilla		
		Winter-green		
		Yeast (baker's/ brewer's)		

Special Variants: *Non-Secretor* BENEFICIAL: bay leaf, yeast (brewer's); AVOID: agar, honey, juniper, maple syrup, rice syrup, sugar (brown/white).

*Do not use if you have high blood pressure.

Herbal Teas

Herbal teas can provide medicinal benefits, and several are SUPER BENEFICIAL for Blood Type AB cardiovascular health. Hawthorn improves coronary function and eases angina. Ginseng helps reduce stress and improve overall cardiac health. Ginger helps reduce the viscosity of blood. Dandelion has mild diuretic effects and is a potassium-rich food.

SUPER BENEFICIAL	BENEFICIAL	NEUTRAL: Allowed Frequently	NEUTRAL: Allowed Infrequently	AVOID
Dandelion	Alfalfa	Catnip	Senna	Aloe
Ginseng	Burdock	Chickweed		Coltsfoot
Hawthorn	Chamomile	Dong quai		Corn silk
Licorice root*	Echinacea	Elder		Fenugreek
Parsley	Ginger	Horehound		Gentian
	Rosehip	Mulberry		Goldenseal
	Strawberry leaf	Peppermint		Hops
		Raspberry leaf		Linden
		Sage		Mullein
		Sarsaparilla		Red clover
		Slippery elm		Rhubarb
		Spearmint		Shepherd's purse
		St. John's wort		Skullcap
		Thyme		
		Valerian		
		Vervain		
		White birch		
		White oak bark		
		Yarrow		
		Yellow dock		
Special Variants: None.				

*Do not use if you have high blood pressure.

Miscellaneous Beverages

You may wish to have a glass of wine occasionally with your meals; you derive substantial benefit to the cardiovascular system from moderate use. Green tea should be part of every Blood Type AB's health plan;

the catechins and polyphenols in green tea have been shown to lower LDL cholesterol by as much as 16 percent. Blood Type AB individuals who are not alcohol sensitive may benefit from the occasional glass of red wine. Researchers have found that red wine increases HDL cholesterol and that HDL particles from wine drinkers were richer in certain components that can play a protective role in cardiovascular disease.

SUPER BENEFICIAL	BENEFICIAL	NEUTRAL: Allowed Frequently	NEUTRAL: Allowed Infrequently	AVOID
Tea (green)	Wine (red)	Seltzer Soda (club) Wine (white)	Beer	Coffee (reg/decaf) Liquor Soda (cola/diet/misc.) Tea, black (reg/decaf)

Special Variants: *Non-Secretor* AVOID: beer.

Supplements

THE BLOOD TYPE AB Diet offers abundant quantities of important nutrients, such as protein and iron. It is important to get as many nutrients as possible from fresh foods and use supplements only to fill in the minor deficiencies in your diet. The following supplement protocols are designed for Blood Type AB individuals who are suffering from cardiovascular disease or related conditions.

Note: If you are being treated for a cardiovascular or related condition, consult your doctor before taking any supplements.

Blood Type AB: Cardiovascular Protection and Enhancement Protocol

Use this protocol for 4–8 weeks, then discontinue for 2 weeks and restart.

SUPPLEMENT	ACTION	DOSAGE
Soy protein powder	Enhances protection of blood vessel lining	Use as directed in a protein drink, once daily
Vitamin C (food derived, from rosehip or acerola cherry)	May help protect against the oxidation of LDL cholesterol by neutralizing free radicals	100–200 mg daily
Garlic	Mild cholesterol-lowering effects	2–4 fresh cloves daily
Lemon juice	Mild blood-thinning ability	Juice of ½ lemon daily
Soluble fiber supplement	Mild cholesterol-lowering effects	3–5 grams daily

Blood Type AB: Specific Cardiovascular Treatment Protocols

Use these protocols for 4–8 weeks, then discontinue for 1 week and restart. Protocols can be combined.

Cholesterol, Triglyceride Control*		
SUPPLEMENT	ACTION	DOSAGE
Guggul gum (*Commiphora mukul*)	Provides vascular support; lowers triglycerides	Standardized for 25 mg guggulsterones of type E and Z. 1 capsule, 1–2 times daily

SUPPLEMENT	ACTION	DOSAGE
Green tea extracts	Reduce low-density lipoprotein cholesterol	1–2 capsules, twice daily. (Formula should contain a minimum of 150 mg of catechins, and 150 mg of other tea antioxidants called polyphenols.)
Pantethine (active vitamin B$_5$)	Lowers cholesterol	500 mg, twice daily

Stress Reduction Protocol

SUPPLEMENT	ACTION	DOSAGE
Chamomile (*Matricaria chamomilla*)	A calming nerve tonic	Herbal tincture; 25 drops in warm water, two to three times daily
L-theanine	Anti-anxiety remedy from green tea	100–200 mg, twice daily
Spreading hogweed (*Boerhaavia diffusa*)	Acts as a stress modifier and a liver protector; lowers cortisol	50–150 mg, twice daily
Holy basil (*Ocimum sanctum*) leaf extract	Lowers cortisol	50 mg, twice daily

Angina Relief Adjunct*

SUPPLEMENT	ACTION	DOSAGE
Coenzyme Q-10 (ubiquinone)	Improves coronary function; reduces angina	30–60 mg daily with meals
L-arginine	Researchers have begun to use arginine in people with angina and congestive heart failure.	1000–2000 mg, twice daily

SUPPLEMENT	ACTION	DOSAGE
Jiaogulan (*Gynostemma pentaphyllum*)	Dramatically decreases the chances of a stroke by inhibiting blood platelets from sticking together, which prevents blood clots from forming. Also prevents artery clogging, reducing heart attack risk. By increasing nitric oxide, a chemical that relaxes blood vessel walls, it increases blood flow. It also reduces cholesterol by about 25%.	50–100 mg, twice daily

Hypertension Control*

SUPPLEMENT	ACTION	DOSAGE
Dandelion (*Taraxacum officinale*)	Mild diuretic, rich in electrolytes	150 mg, twice daily
L-arginine	Mild to moderate effects on high blood pressure; increases nitric oxide production, which relaxes artery walls	1000–2000 mg, twice daily
Magnesium	May help relax arteries, resulting in slight decrease in blood pressure; mild blood-clot-inhibiting effects, produces mild improvement in angina	250–500 mg, once or twice daily

Homocysteine Control or enhancement of blood flow*		
SUPPLEMENT	**ACTION**	**DOSAGE**
Folic acid	Lowers homocysteine and builds blood	400 mcg, twice daily
Vitamin B$_{12}$ (methylcobalamine)	Works with folic acid to help metabolize homocysteine	1000 mcg daily
Pyridoxine (vitamin B$_6$)	Works with folic acid to help metabolize homocysteine	50 mg, twice daily
Fish oils	May slow development of heart disease resulting from increased LDL. Omega-3 fatty acids in fish oils discourage platelets from clumping.	1000 mg, once or twice daily

*Check with your doctor before beginning this or any other nutritional protocol, especially if you are currently taking prescription medication.

The Exercise Component

FOR BLOOD TYPE AB, overall fitness is achieved with a balance of moderate aerobic activity and mentally soothing, stress-reducing exercises. Below is a list of exercises that are recommended for Blood Type AB.

EXERCISE	**DURATION**	**FREQUENCY**
Martial arts	30–60 minutes	2–3 x week
Cycling	45–60 minutes	2–3 x week
Hiking	30–60 minutes	2–3 x week
Golf (no cart!)	60–90 minutes	2–3 x week
Walking	40–50 minutes	2–3 x week
Pilates	40–50 minutes	2–3 x week

EXERCISE	DURATION	FREQUENCY
Swimming	45 minutes	2–3 x week
Yoga	40–50 minutes	1–2 x week
T'ai Chi	40–50 minutes	1–2 x week

3 Steps to Effective Exercise

1. Warm up with stretching and flexibility moves, before you start your aerobic exercise.
2. To achieve maximum cardiovascular benefits, work toward an elevated heart rate that is about 70 percent of your capacity. Once you reach the elevated rate, continue exercising to maintain that rate for twenty to thirty minutes. To calculate your maximum heart rate and performance level:
   - Subtract your age from 220.
   - Multiply the difference by .70 (or .60 if you are over age sixty). This is the high end of your performance.
   - Multiply the remainder by .50. This is the low end of your performance.
3. Finish each aerobic session with at least a five-minute cooldown of stretching and relaxation moves.

Getting Started: The First Month

IF YOU ARE NEW to the Blood Type Diet, the following guidelines will introduce you to the Blood Type AB regimen over a period of one month. Follow these recommendations as closely as possible, using a journal to record your personal experiences with the diet. In addition to factors that are measurable in medical tests (EKG, cholesterol levels, blood pressure, cardiac stress tests), take the time to note changes in your energy levels, sleep patterns, digestion, and overall well-being.

Blood Type AB Cardiovascular Diet Checklist

Derive your protein primarily from sources other than red meat. ☐
Low levels of hydrochloric acid and intestinal alkaline phosphatase make it difficult for Blood Type AB to digest meats.

Use soy foods and seafood as your primary protein. ☐

Include regular portions of richly oiled cold-water fish every ☐
week.

Include modest amounts of cultured dairy foods in your diet, ☐
but limit fresh milk products, which cause excess mucus production.

Don't overdo the grains, especially wheat-derived foods. ☐
Avoid wheat if you have heart disease.

Eat lots of BENEFICIAL fruits and vegetables, especially those ☐
high in antioxidants and fiber.

Avoid coffee. Substitute green tea every day for extra cardio- ☐
vascular and immune system benefits.

Week 1

Blood Type Diet and Supplements

- Eliminate your most harmful AVOID foods—chicken, corn, buckwheat, most shellfish, and lectin-activated beans.

- Avoid wheat if you have heart disease, diabetes, or are overweight. For example, have soy-based foods 5 times and omega-3-rich fish 3 to 4 times, with lots of BENEFICIAL vegetables and fruit.

- Incorporate at least 1 SUPER BENEFICIAL food into your daily diet. For example, eat slices of fresh pineapple over yogurt, or sprinkle walnuts on a salad.

- If you're a coffee drinker, begin to wean yourself by cutting your daily consumption in half. Substitute green tea or one of the SUPER BENEFICIAL herbal teas.

Exercise Regimen

- Plan to exercise at least 4 days this week, for 45 minutes each day.

  2 days: walking or light aerobic activity

  2 days: yoga or T'ai Chi

- If you experience angina during exercise, consult with a physician. Angina is a warning sign that some of your heart muscle is not getting enough oxygen.

- Use your journal to detail the time, activity, distance, and amount of weight. Note the number of repetitions for each exercise.

■ WEEK 1 SUCCESS STRATEGY ■
Chi Breathing

Chi breathing is based on the Taoist concept of Chi Gong, which represents energy as flowing according to certain routes in your body. Positive release is accessible through refining the breath. The calming, stress-relieving effects of this exercise are remarkable. It can be performed by anyone, regardless of age, fitness, or medical condition.

1. Stand comfortably, feet shoulder-width apart, knees slightly bent, arms at your side. Relax your neck and shoulder muscles and focus on your solar plexus (center of the body). It is okay to sway a bit—that's normal.

2. Start to rock back and forth gently. Inhale deeply as you rock forward onto the balls of your feet; exhale as you rock backward onto your heels.

3. As you inhale, lift your relaxed arms up and forward, keeping them relaxed and slightly bent. As you exhale, let your arms float down. Imagine that your hands are pulsing around an imaginary ball of energy.

4. Repeat, gradually refining the rhythm and developing the ability to "drop" your breath from the lungs to the solar plexus.

5. Repeat four to five times, then relax, letting your hands drop to your sides and closing your eyes. Concentrate on feeling relaxed and centered.

Week 2

Blood Type Diet and Supplements

- Begin to eliminate the next level of AVOID foods—grains, vegetables, and fruits—that react poorly with Type AB blood.
- Eat 2 to 3 BENEFICIAL proteins every day.
- Continue to incorporate SUPER BENEFICIAL foods into your daily diet.
- Choose the NEUTRAL foods listed as Allowed Frequently, over those listed as Allowed Infrequently.
- If you're a coffee drinker, continue to cut your coffee intake, replacing it with BENEFICIAL herbal teas. Drink a cup of green tea every morning.
- Manage your mealtimes to aid proper digestion. Avoid eating on the run. Make your meals relaxing, sit-down affairs. Eat slowly and chew thoroughly to encourage digestive secretions.

Exercise Regimen

- Continue to exercise at least 4 days this week, for 45 minutes each day.

  2 days: walking or light aerobic activity

  2 days: yoga or T'ai Chi
- If your work is sedentary, get in the habit of taking a couple of "movement" breaks during the day. Walk around the block or up and down stairs.

■ **WEEK 2 SUCCESS STRATEGY** ■
Heart-Healthy Alternatives

There's no need to feel deprived on the Blood Type Diet. Satisfy your cravings with these alternatives:

INSTEAD OF...		EAT...
processed sweets	→ → →	pineapple slices or raisins
salty foods	→ → →	nori (seaweed) or celery sticks
ice cream	→ → →	frozen fruit ice or sorbet
fatty foods	→ → →	walnuts, or peanuts
creamy foods	→ → →	vegetable puree, with 1 tblsp olive oil and 1 tblsp soy lecithin

Week 3

Blood Type Diet and Supplements

- When you plan your meals for week 3, choose BENEFICIAL foods to replace NEUTRAL foods whenever possible.
- Eliminate all remaining AVOID foods.
- Liberally incorporate SUPER BENEFICIAL foods into your daily diet.
- Completely wean yourself from coffee, substituting green tea or herbal tea.

Exercise Regimen

- Continue to exercise at least 4 days this week, for 45 minutes each day.

  2 days: walking or light aerobic activity

  2 days: yoga or T'ai Chi

■ WEEK 3 SUCCESS STRATEGY ■
Timing Is Everything

For Blood Type AB, the timing of your meals can be almost as important as what you eat. This is particularly true if you're trying to lose weight. The following are helpful guidelines:

- Never skip meals. You won't be "saving" calories, as the metabolic reaction will foil your efforts.
- Make breakfast your most important protein-rich meal of the day. The result will be an efficient metabolism all day long.
- Vary your meal sizes: big breakfast, medium lunch, small dinner.
- Resist the late-night munchies, but if you have problems regulating blood sugar, have a small protein snack—yogurt or soy milk—before bedtime.

Week 4

Blood Type Diet

- Continue at the week 3 level, focusing on BENEFICIAL and SUPER BENEFICIAL foods.

Exercise Regimen

- Continue at the week 3 level.

- Review your progress, noting in your journal improvements in strength and flexibility. Determine which exercise regimen has worked for you, including time of day, setting, and activity level.

■ WEEK 4 SUCCESS STRATEGY ■
Think Yourself Healthy

Take advantage of Blood Type AB's natural ability to relieve stress through meditation or guided imagery. I've never medicated Type AB individuals who have high blood pressure without first teaching them some simple visualization techniques and sending them home to try them out for a few weeks. Those that did almost never required medication.

Here is a very simple visualization exercise to help control high blood pressure. Do this visualization two to four times daily for five to eight minutes.

Find a quiet place, and make yourself comfortable and relaxed. Close your eyes and let your arms and hands lie limply at your sides or in your lap. Take a few deep breaths, inhaling through your nose and exhaling through your mouth, while imagining the red blood cells of your circulatory system coursing through your arteries and veins. See them slipping and sliding along the walls, which periodically open up like Venetian blinds to allow cells to move from the inside of the arteries out and from the outside in. Imagine the walls of your arteries relaxing and bending. Now expand the image and visualize your entire body. See the blood circulating from your heart to the arteries, to the capillaries, to the veins, then back to the lungs and heart.

A Final Word

IN SUMMARY, the secret to fighting cardiovascular disease with the Blood Type AB Diet involves:

1. Increasing active tissue mass (calorie-burning tissue) by eating a diet rich in soy protein, healthy seafood, and green vegetables.
2. Minimizing consumption of the insulin-mimicking lectins abundant in AVOID beans, grains, and vegetables, which can contribute to metabolic syndrome, a precursor to heart disease.
3. Improving your metabolic health, lowering your cholesterol, controlling your blood pressure, improving liver function, and lowering your risk for heart disease by limiting your consumption of high-fat foods.
4. Using supplements intelligently to block the effect of insulin-mimicking lectins, provide antioxidant support, and protect delicate nerve tissue from destruction.
5. Working on the mind/body connection to enhance your ability to control biologic functions through modalities such as meditation and imagery.

Appendices

A Simple
Definition
of Terms

agglutination: Clumping, or "gluing," together. One means by which the immune system defends against foreign matter and toxins, notably against lectins and opposing blood type material.

aneurysm: A weakening and possible rupture of a blood vessel or arterial wall. Aneurysms can go undetected for years, and when they erupt they can be fatal.

angina pectoris: A recurring pain or discomfort in the chest that occurs when some part of the heart does not receive enough blood. It is a common symptom of coronary heart disease, which occurs when vessels that carry blood to the heart become narrowed and blocked due to atherosclerosis.

antibody: The product of the immune system when it is stimulated by specific antigens. There are many classes of antibodies, among them "agglutinins," which isolate foreign substances by clumping them together so that they may be eliminated. Blood Types O, A, and B manufacture antibodies to other blood types. Blood Type AB, the universal recipient, manufactures no antibodies to other blood types.

antigen: A chemical that provokes an immune system antibody response. The blood type "I.D." present on the blood cells, identified as Type A or B, is one example. A Type AB cell has both of these antigens. The blood type having no antigen is described as O—or "Zero." As we age, it is to our advantage to shore up our store of circulating anti–blood type antigens, as lower levels mean increased susceptibility to diseases arising from substances and organisms bearing opposing antigens.

antioxidant: Antioxidants are important, naturally occurring nutrients that help maintain health by slowing the destructive aging process of cellular molecules such as free radicals. As cells function normally in the body, they produce damaged molecules, called free radicals. Antioxidants help prevent widespread cellular destruction by willingly donating components to stabilize free radicals. Many healthy foods are rich sources of antioxidants, including the element selenium and the vitamins C, E, and A.

atherosclerosis: A slow, progressive disease involving damage to the arterial walls from the buildup of fats, cholesterol, fibrin, platelets, cellular debris, and calcium. These substances can stimulate the cells of the arterial wall to produce still other substances that result in further accumulation of cells, causing atherosclerotic lesions, called plaque. Plaque may partially or totally block the blood's flow through an artery, causing bleeding into the plaque or formation of a blood clot (thrombus) on the plaque's surface. If either of these occurs and blocks the entire artery, a heart attack or stroke (brain attack) may result.

atrial arrhythmia: A disturbance in the heart rhythm caused by irregular contractions of the heart muscle.

biomarker: The biochemical predictor of physiological events (such as cancer or a long life). William Evans and Irwin Rosenberg coined the term to describe those aspects of physical function upon which healthier aging particularly depends. Basal metabolic rate (influenced by proportionate muscle mass), aerobic capacity, strength, blood sugar tolerance, body fat percentage, and bone density together provide a reliable indication of one's "biological age," or the health of the total physical system.

blood type: The term commonly used to refer to the ABO blood group system. Originally used primarily to determine suitable blood and organ donor–recipient matches, ABO type determines many of the digestive and immunological characteristics of the body, as well as susceptibility to the diseases arising from infection, immune suppression, and digestive impairment. It is also one of the tools of anthropology in establishing the origins, socioeconomic development, and movements of ancient peoples.

carbohydrate intolerance: A condition in which simple carbohydrate foods, such as starch and sugar, are not easily or fully digested. Due to the more acidic stomach environment of Blood Types O and B, these carbohydrates remain overlong in the digestive system, leading to a toxic bowel, higher body fat, and prolonged overproduction of insulin and elevated triglycerides. Given sufficient quantities of carbohydrates in the diet, an individual of any blood type may develop this intolerance.

cerebrovascular accident: A stroke, or brain attack, caused by the buildup of plaque. A piece of plaque becomes dislodged and gets stuck in the circulation to the brain, causing a stroke. Some are massive and fatal, while others are considered mini-strokes, or transient ischemic attacks.

cholesterol: A fatlike steroid alcohol found in animal tissue, especially the brain, nerve fiber sheaths, liver, kidneys, and adrenal glands. Approximately 90 percent of the body's cholesterol is produced by the liver, with the remaining amount obtained from the diet. High blood cholesterol, especially the levels of LDL (low-density lipoprotein) and VLDL (very low-density lipoprotein), is associated most strongly in Blood Types A and AB with the development of heart disease. Studies have found high HDL cholesterol levels, regardless of total serum cholesterol, predictive of long life.

claudication: The pain in the calf or thigh muscle that occurs after walking a certain distance, such as a block or two, and which ceases with rest. Claudication occurs when a narrowed artery prevents adequate blood flow to a muscle.

congestive heart failure: Any condition that disturbs the pumping of blood through the heart muscle and throughout the body, or prevents blood from oxygenating the lungs.

high-density lipoprotein (HDL): With LDL and VLDL, responsible for the transport of cholesterol and fats in the bloodstream. HDL is the "good" lipoprotein (fat/protein) of the cholesterol trio. Relatively high HDL levels (over 60 mg/dL) have been correlated with a lower risk for heart disease, especially in women.

hypertension: Persistently high arterial blood pressure, often without noticeable symptoms; a risk factor for the development of heart disease, kidney disease, and stroke.

hyperthyroidism: The overactive thyroid is conventionally treated with long-term antithyroid drugs or partial removal or destruction with radioactive iodine or surgery. Thyroid diseases show a preference for Blood Type O individuals. While medical intervention is recommended in the case of hyperthyroid function, reducing the types and amount of anti–blood type lectins present in the diet, especially those found in certain grains and legumes, can be of great help in resolving these conditions.

hypoglycemia: Low blood glucose levels. Symptoms include nausea, weakness, dizziness, and cold sweat. Hypoglycemia can be resolved through the use of appropriate protein foods and the avoidance of deleterious lectins, refined starches, and sugar.

hypothyroidism: Underproduction of thyroid hormone, thyroxine (t3) and/or free triiodothyronine (t4)), conventionally treated by hormone replacement therapy. Thyroid conditions often respond favorably to a blood type–appropriate diet.

insulin: A polypeptide hormone secreted by the beta cells of the islets of Langerhans in the pancreas to reduce high blood sugar levels. Inappropriate diet can trigger defective insulin response, leading to fatigue, overweight, and the development of diabetes mellitus and other metabolic dysfunctions, as well as magnifying the effects of estrogen.

insulin resistance: The condition in which insulinlike lectins, bound to fat molecules' insulin receptors, signal the fat cells to continue to store rather than release the fats for fuel. Triglyceride conversion is impaired, resulting in a sluggish metabolic rate that promotes further fat storage. Non-secretors particularly, and individuals with grain- and sugar-based diets generally, have a greater risk of developing insulin resistance.

intestinal alkaline phosphatase (IAP): An enzyme manufactured in the small intestine, involved in the breakdown of dietary proteins and fats, including cholesterol, and in the assimilation of calcium. In Blood Types O and B, animal protein meals stimulate IAP production levels, thereby lowering blood cholesterol levels and improving calcium absorption. Blood Type O secretors typically have the highest IAP response, followed by Blood Type B secretors.

There is evidence that the A antigen possessed by Types A and AB acts to bind, or neutralize, nearly all of the little IAP they produce.

ischemia: Insufficient supply of blood to an organ, usually caused by a blocked artery. Myocardial ischemia is inadequate blood flow to the heart, usually as a result of coronary artery blockage.

lectins: Proteins that attach to preferred receptors in the human body. Food lectins are often blood type–specific. A lectin's action may initiate agglutination, inflammation, abnormal proliferation of cells of the immune and nervous systems, or insulin resistance, depending upon the type of cells targeted. Abundant in the vegetable kingdom, lectins are fewer in number and type among animal foods, such as eggs, fish, and meats.

low-density lipoprotein (LDL): The "bad" lipoprotein (fat/protein), which acts, with HDL and VLDL, as a carrier for cholesterol and fats in the bloodstream. While small quantities are necessary, less than 100 mg/dL is desirable, 130 to 159 mg/dL is borderline high, and over 160 is a positive risk factor for the development of heart disease and atherosclerosis.

metabolic syndrome (formerly Syndrome X): The name given to a cluster of metabolic dysfunctions: insulin resistance and obesity, accompanied by elevated blood-sugar, blood pressure, triglycerides and LDL cholesterol, and low HDL cholesterol. This group of conditions is a precursor to the onset of type 2 diabetes, heart disease, and atherosclerosis.

metabolism: The aggregate of physical and chemical processes by which organisms maintain life, in the opposing functions of building tissue (anabolism) and breaking down tissue and foreign matter to be used as fuel (catabolism).

myocardial infarction: A heart attack.

stenosis: Hardening of the arteries.

thrombosis: A condition in which a blood clot forms, travels through the circulatory system, and finally lodges somewhere.

triglycerides: The body's fat stores, also present in the bloodstream, largely composed of glycerol esters of saturated fatty acids. They are an important source of energy for the heart muscle. Elevated triglycerides are a risk factor for heart disease and stroke, especially in association with high LDL cholesterol and/or insulin resistance.

type 1 diabetes: A condition that occurs when the pancreas is unable to produce insulin. It usually begins in childhood or young adulthood and lasts throughout a diabetic's life. Type 1 accounts for about 10 percent of all diabetes cases.

type 2 diabetes: A condition involving the insufficient production or the poor utilization of insulin, which delivers glucose to the body's cells.

ventricular arrhythmia: A disturbance of the electrical rhythm of the more muscular of the heart's pumping stations, the one that distributes blood throughout the rest of the body.

very low-density lipoprotein (VLDL): A lipoprotein (fat/protein) substance that carries cholesterol and fats, including triglycerides, through the bloodstream. VLDL is considered the "worst" form of cholesterol, as fairly low amounts are associated with increased risk of heart disease and atherosclerosis.

FAQs: Blood Type and Cardiovascular Disease

FAQs: Blood Type O and Cardiovascular Disease

I have been on the Blood Type O diet before and loved it. I want to start again, but I can't seem to get through the first few days that it takes for me to get over the obsessive cravings, especially to wheat. Any suggestions?

Many Blood Type Os report having a rough time adjusting to the loss of wheat in the diet, especially in the first few weeks. I've found that the use of the amino acid glutamine can help offset these feelings until the Type O Diet begins to help up-regulate your dopamine levels.

In the brain, glutamine is converted to glutamic acid, the only alternate source of glucose available to the brain. It provides a ready

source of brain fuel for hypoglycemics and helps stave off sugar cravings and hypoglycemic symptoms that develop when blood-sugar levels drop too low.

Glutamine is also an important source of energy for the nervous
system. If the brain is not receiving enough glucose, it compensates by
increasing glutamine metabolism for energy—hence the popular per-
ception of glutamine as "brain food" and its use as a pick-me-up. Glutamine users often report more energy, less fatigue, and better mood.

Glutamine is plentiful in both animal and plant protein. The typical American diet provides between 3.5 and 7 grams of glutamine;
more is synthesized according to need. Even so, heavy stress, such as
strenuous exercise, infectious disease, surgery, or other acute trauma,
leads to glutamine depletion with consequent immune dysfunction,
intestinal problems, and muscle wasting. Consequently, it has been
proposed that glutamine should be classified as a "conditionally essential amino acid." A useful dose is 500 to 750 mg in powder or cap-
sule form between meals for a week or two. By the way, glutamine
(unlike most amino acids) is rather pleasant tasting, with a slightly
sweet flavor.

**I am a fifty-five-year-old Blood Type O woman with a long history
of recurrent major depression. Your suggestion to exercise vigorously rather than just walking has improved my sense of well-
being. My naturopath has also recommended St. John's wort. Why
do you discourage this supplement for Blood Type O?**

Blood Type O has lower levels of the enzyme MAO, and St. John's
wort is an MAO inhibitor. This may explain why many Type O individuals on St. John's wort say they feel "weird" or have disturbing
dreams. I have found, however, that Blood Type Os with mild to moderate depression benefit from the amino acid tyrosine, which can boost
dopamine levels, or the Russian adaptogenic herb Rhodiola, which
helps modulate adrenaline and dopamine levels in the brain. Studies
have shown that in men with recent heart attacks, those who were
Type O tested much higher on the scale of so-called "type A behav-
ior" than the other blood types. This makes the goal of eliminating excess adrenaline even more important.

I've read that too much protein can cause calcium loss. Should people on the Type O or Type B Diet be concerned about osteoporosis?

Protein-related calcium loss may occur for Blood Type A non-secretors who have the lowest levels of intestinal alkaline phosphatase, an enzyme made by the intestine to split dietary fat and help assimilate calcium. However, Blood Types O and B have high levels of this enzyme. This is yet another example of the adage "One man's food is another man's poison." For Blood Types O and B, the adoption of a high-protein diet will support healthier bones.

I am Type O, and I've been taking a supplement of whey protein with milk to help increase muscle mass. I also consume four egg whites a day for protein. Can you give me an alternative?

I suggest you switch to an albumin-based protein and use rice or almond milk instead of dairy. Keep in mind, though, that the best way for Blood Type O to increase muscle mass is with a high-protein diet and intensive aerobic and strength-building exercise.

FAQs: Blood Type A and Cardiovascular Disease

Will a macrobiotic diet work for Blood Type A?

Macrobiotics can work for Blood Type A, though you will have to make adjustments for specific foods that have problematic lectin effects for you. Examples include kidney and lima beans, honeydew melon, and corn oil. I would also place more emphasis on omega-3-rich seafoods and plenty of soy.

I have what the doctors say is the beginning of congestive heart failure. What can I do that is not drug related?

Hawthorn extract is beneficial in the treatment of chronic heart failure, according to a new review published in the *American Journal of Medicine.* I've found it to be helpful for Blood Types A, B, and AB, in maintaining cardiovascular health. Hawthorn is one of the most popular medicinal herbs in the United States and Europe. The leaves, flowers, and berries of the hawthorn tree (*Crataegus* spp.) have been used historically to treat ailments of the cardiovascular system. Extracts have demonstrated antioxidant and anti-inflammatory activities and the ability to dilate blood vessels, including those supplying the heart. Studies show that hawthorn can improve the function of the heart muscle, increase blood flow to the heart, lower blood pressure, promote regular heart rhythm, and lower cholesterol levels. Hawthorn can also improve the symptoms of heart failure such as fatigue and shortness of breath. Other supplements that I have used successfully are the amino acid taurine and the element zinc. Check the Blood Type A cardiovascular protocol for the proper dosage. As always, make certain that you have discussed supplement options with your physician.

My husband is Blood Type A, and he has high blood pressure and minor arterial damage. Is coenzyme Q-10 a good supplement for him to take?

Studies have shown that supplementation with coenzyme Q-10 can be effective in the treatment of cardiovascular diseases such as congestive heart failure, cardiac arrhythmias, and hypertension. Based on its safety and apparent efficacy, the use of coenzyme Q-10, in combination with conventional medications, can be recommended for the treatment of cardiovascular disease. Since Blood Type A has a high risk for cardiovascular disease, it would appear that taking supplemental coenzyme Q-10 would be advisable, especially if you are a non-secretor. A typical dose can range from 30 to 100 mg daily. Other blood types may benefit from coenzyme Q-10 supplementation as well, although I use it more frequently for Blood Type A patients.

One caveat: Without a small amount of lipid (fat) in the gut, the absorption of coenzyme Q-10 is virtually nil. To ensure proper assimilation, take it with the largest meal of the day.

I have a Blood Type A friend diagnosed with vasculitis. I'm helping her begin using the Type A food lists. What herbs or other supplements might be beneficial as she begins changing her diet?

Vasculitis is a general term for a group of diseases that involve inflammation in blood vessels. Blood vessels of all sizes may be affected, from the largest vessel in the body (the aorta) to the smallest blood vessels in the skin. The size of the blood vessel affected varies according to the specific type of vasculitis. It is clear that the immune system plays a critical role in the tissue damage caused by vasculitis. The immune system, normally a protective organ of the body, becomes hyperactive in vasculitis because of some unknown stimulus, leading to inflammation within the body's tissues. Inflammation in blood vessel walls leads to narrowing of the vessels. The resulting reduction of blood supply to a particular tissue or organ causes damage. Therapies I've used in combination with diet to help heal vasculitis include:

- Bromelain, the enzyme from pineapple, has both clot-dissolving and anti-inflammatory properties.
- Ganoderma mushroom is often used in traditional Chinese medicine to treat vasculitis.
- Antioxidants, such as vitamin E and glutathione, have been shown to be effective in helping to regulate oxidative stress on the blood vessel wall. One of the best ways to raise intracellular glutathione is the herb milk thistle.
- The B vitamin folic acid is quite effective at lowering homocysteine levels. Quite a bit of evidence suggests that lowering homocysteine levels can help control vasculitis.

I am Blood Type A, and I have a condition called intermittent claudication. Would eating right for my blood type be of any value?

Intermittent claudication (IC) occurs when the leg muscles do not receive the oxygen-rich blood required during exercise, causing an aching pain, cramping, tightness, or fatigue in the thigh, calf, or buttock. IC is definitely associated with blood type, and Type A has the highest rate of occurrence. Following the diet for Blood Type A and using the protocols specific for cholesterol reduction is an excellent start toward getting the condition under control.

FAQs: Blood Type B and Cardiovascular Disease

I am Blood Type B, and I just had angioplasty. Is there anything I can do to reduce the risk of a repeat?

In a study of people who underwent artery-clearing angioplasty, a course of B vitamins following the procedure significantly reduced the risk of needing a repeat procedure. Everyone should make sure that they are getting their B vitamins, especially if you have a heart condition.

I have been on the Type B Diet for several months, and I've lost over twenty pounds. But I'm having trouble overcoming my sugar cravings.

Sugar cravings are usually a sign that your liver is having trouble adjusting to the new way of eating and needs some rehabilitation. Try taking the herb milk thistle and drinking a cup of licorice root tea at about 10:00 A.M. and 2:00 P.M. (Do not use licorice without physician supervision if you suffer from high blood pressure.)

I followed a diet very close to the Type B Diet for many years. Then I had a heart attack, and my physicians put me on a vegan (Type A) diet. I have lost 60 pounds, but my cholesterol has gone up. I'm concerned about the amount of saturated fat on a Type B diet.

If you eat lean, organic meats and exercise properly, you should have no problem with saturated fat. By the way, an increase in cholesterol is not uncommon for Type B vegans. It is probably a response to excess insulin production. Hyperinsulinemia has twice the risk factor for heart disease as elevated cholesterol and would be much more of a threat to you.

Why are sprouted grains allowed for Blood Types O and B but not wheat? What's the difference? Can I eat commercially made sprouted grain breads?

"Ezekiel 4:9" and "Essene" (manna) breads are made from 100 percent sprouted grains, as opposed to all other commercially available sprouted grain breads, which also have regular flour included in the recipe. The lectins in many grains are contained in the seed coat. The seed coat is actually metabolized by the seed/grain when it is germinated, thereby eliminating the lectin and rendering the food usable. New brand names of sprouted grain bread are continually coming to market. Always check the ingredient label on the commercial Ezekiel 4:9 breads for the presence of unsprouted flour or grain.

A friend of mine combines the Blood Type Diet with another popular diet, and she has lost a lot of weight. What do you think about this?

If you really want to combine another diet with the right diet for your blood type, follow the Type B Diet as your primary food selection plan and use it as a basis for judging elements in the second diet. Overall, this is just extra hard work, since the diet for your blood type is by far more specific to you than the popular one-size-fits-all diets. A second diet plan may specify certain times to eat, carbohydrate-to-protein ratios, amounts of fat, or other criteria. Just try to stay away from the blood type "avoids," and eat lots of SUPER BENEFICIAL foods.

FAQs: Blood Type AB and Cardiovascular Disease

How problematic is the mineral-blocking action of phytic acid in soy?

Soy—especially the bran or hulls—has been vilified by some as "anti-nutrient." This is due to the presence of phytates, compounds capable of binding calcium, magnesium, zinc, and iron in the intestines and preventing their absorption. As with most nutrition issues, one should seek to evaluate both sides of the controversy, keeping in mind the great advantage provided by our understanding of blood type variations. As I always like to remind people during these "good food/bad food" arguments, one person's food can be another person's poison.

In a normal Type AB Diet, in which soy is not the sole dependent source for amino acids, the negative effects are minimal. The benefits, however, can be tremendous. Because phytates bind excess iron, which can promote free radical DNA damage in the colon, soy foods can reduce this local oxidative damage. Phytates in plant fiber are also associated with reductions in the incidence of colon cancer and directly reduce serum cholesterol and triglycerides, a partial risk factor for atherosclerosis. Phytates prevent absorption of excess iron in its most reactive form. Excess iron systemically leads to oxidative stress, which is implicated in heart disease, diabetes, arthritis, and cancer.

The bottom line: If you were a lab animal being fed nothing but soy husks for several weeks, you would see a drop in your mineral levels. If you are a Blood Type AB individual looking to minimize your risk of certain degenerative diseases by adding a rational amount of soy to your otherwise well-balanced diet, it's a good thing.

Should I avoid genetically engineered foods on the Blood Type Diet?

Yes! Genetic engineering moves lectin molecules from one species to another. Since lectins are the molecules that interact with our blood types, an acceptable food can easily become unacceptable with genetic engineering. Currently, the only way to safely avoid genetically engineered foods is to choose organic.

I'm Blood Type AB and my wife is Blood Type O. What blood types will our children be?

The offspring of Blood Type O–Blood Type AB parents will either be Blood Type A or Blood Type B, as both the A and B alleles are dominant to the *o* allele. However, your child will possess a recessive *o* allele (in addition to their dominant allele), which they may pass on to their own offspring, and use to produce Blood Type O offspring.

Resources
and Products

General

American Heart Association
7272 Greenville Avenue
Dallas, TX 75231
1-800-AHA-USA-1 (1-800-242-8721)
www.americanheart.org

A national voluntary health agency whose mission is to reduce disability and death from cardiovascular diseases and stroke.

American Stroke Association
National Center
7272 Greenville Avenue
Dallas, TX 75231
1-888-4-STROKE (1-888-478-7653)
www.strokeassociation.org

The American Stroke Association is the division of the American Heart Association that's solely focused on reducing disability and death from stroke through research, education, fund-raising, and advocacy.

WomenHeart
818 18th Street, NW
Suite 730
Washington, DC 20006
202-728-7199
www.womenheart.org

WomenHeart is the only national patient advocacy organization founded by women with heart disease and dedicated to reducing death and disability among the 8 million American women living with heart disease.

American Diabetes Association
1701 N. Beauregard Street
Alexandria, VA 22311
1-800-DIABETES (1-800-342-2383)
www.diabetes.org

The nation's leading nonprofit organization for diabetes research, information, and advocacy.

Nutrition Research

The Institute for Human Individuality
Southwest College of Naturopathic Medicine
2140 E. Broadway Road
Tempe, AZ 85282
480-858-9100
www.ifhi-online.org

The Institute for Human Individuality is under the 501c3 status of Southwest College of Naturopathic Medicine. Its primary goal is to foster research in the expanding area of human nutrigenomics. Nutrigenomics seeks to provide a molecular understanding of how common dietary chemicals affect health by altering the expression or structure of an individual's genetic makeup.

Products

To purchase supplements mentioned in this book or suggested by your naturopathic physician, your local health-food store is always an excellent resource

Blood Type–Specific Resources

Dr. Peter D'Adamo

The D'Adamo Naturopathic Center in Stamford, Connecticut, blends time-honored natural healing techniques with state-of-the-art diagnostics. The clinic staff is comprised of naturopathic physicians (NDs) working with medical doctors (MDs), nurses (RNs), and other licensed health professionals, all under the precepts and guidance of Dr. Peter D'Adamo. To find out more or to schedule an appointment, please contact:

The D'Adamo Naturopathic Center
2009 Summer Street
Stamford, CT 06905
203-348-4800

www.dadamo.com
The World Wide Web has proven to be a valuable venue for exploring and applying the tenets of the Blood Type Diet and lifestyle. Since January 1997, hundreds of thousands have visited the site to participate in the ABO chat groups, peruse the scientific archives, share experiences and recipes, and learn more about the science of blood type.

Blood Type Specialty Products
and Supplements

NORTH AMERICAN PHARMACAL, INC., is the official distributor of Blood Type Specialty Products. The product line includes supplements, books, tapes, teas, meal replacement bars, cosmetics, and support material that make eating and living right for your type easier.

North American Pharmacal, Inc.
12 High Street
Norwalk, CT 06851
203-866-7664
Toll free: 877-ABO TYPE (877-226-8973)
Fax: 203-838-4066
www.4yourtype.com

Home Blood-Typing Kits

North American Pharmacal, Inc., is the official distributor of Home Blood Type Testing Kits. Each kit costs $9.95 (plus shipping and handling) and is a single-use, disposable, educational device capable of determining one individual's ABO and Rhesus (Rh) blood type. Results are obtained within about four to five minutes. If you have several friends or family members who need to learn their blood type, you will need to order a separate home blood-typing kit for each individual.

The Blood Type Library

The following books are available in bookstores, health-food stores, selected grocery and specialty stores, on the Web, and through North American Pharmacal.

Eat Right 4 Your Type
The Individualized Diet Solution to Staying Healthy, Living Longer, and Achieving Your Ideal Weight

Dr. Peter J. D'Adamo, with Catherine Whitney
G. P. Putnam's Sons, 1996
   The original Blood Type Diet ® book, with over 2 million copies sold in more than sixty-five languages.

Cook Right 4 Your Type
The Practical Kitchen Companion to Eat Right 4 Your Type
Dr. Peter J. D'Adamo, with Catherine Whitney
G. P. Putnam's Sons, 1998 (Berkley Trade Paperback, 1999)
   Includes over 200 original recipes, thirty-day meal plans, and guidelines for each blood type.

Live Right 4 Your Type
The Individualized Prescription for Maximizing Health, Metabolism, and Vitality in Every Stage of Your Life
Dr. Peter J. D'Adamo, with Catherine Whitney
G. P. Putnam's Sons, 2001
   A total health and lifestyle plan based on the individual variations observed for each blood type. Includes new research on the mind-body connection and the importance of blood type secretor status.

Eat Right 4 Your Type Complete Blood Type Encyclopedia
Dr. Peter J. D'Adamo, with Catherine Whitney
Riverhead Books, 2002
   The A–Z reference guide for the blood type connection to symptoms, disease, conditions, medications, vitamins, supplements, herbs, and food.

4 Your Type Pocket Guides
Blood Type, Food, Beverage and Supplement Lists
Peter J. D'Adamo, with Catherine Whitney
Berkley Books, 2002
   The Eat Right 4 Your Type Portable and Personal Blood Type Guides are pocket-sized and user-friendly. They serve as a handy reference tool while shopping, cooking, and eating out. Each book contains the food, beverage, and supplement list for each blood type plus handy tips and ideas for incorporating the blood type diet into your daily life.

Eat Right 4 Your Baby
The Individualized Guide to Fertility and Maximum Health During Pregnancy, Nursing, and Your Baby's First Year
Dr. Peter J. D'Adamo, with Catherine Whitney
G. P. Putnam's Sons, 2003

An invaluable guide for couples looking to combine the best of naturopathic and blood type science to maximize the health of mother and baby—with practical blood type–specific guidelines for achieving a healthy state before pregnancy, eating and living right during pregnancy, and how to continue in good health during baby's first year.

Dr. Peter J. D'Adamo's Eat Right 4 Your Type Health Library
Diabetes: Fight It with the Blood Type Diet ®
Cancer: Fight It with the Blood Type Diet ®
Cardiovascular Disease: Fight It with the Blood Type Diet ®

Index